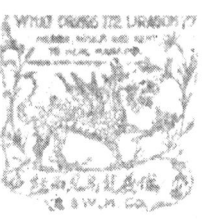

THE SCIENCE OF ORIENTAL MEDICINE DIET AND HYGIENE

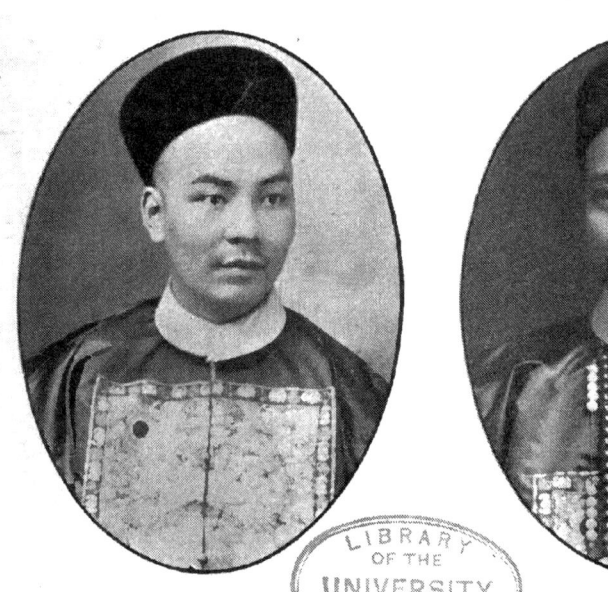

TOM LEONG

Vice-President of the FOO & WING HERB COMPANY, a valued member of this progressive and influential incorporation, also a graduate of the Imperial Medical College at Pekin.

T. FOO YUEN

President of the FOO & WING HERB COMPANY, Ex-Official Physician to the Emperor of China, graduate of the Imperial Medical College at Pekin, widely known from his long and successful business career in Southern California.

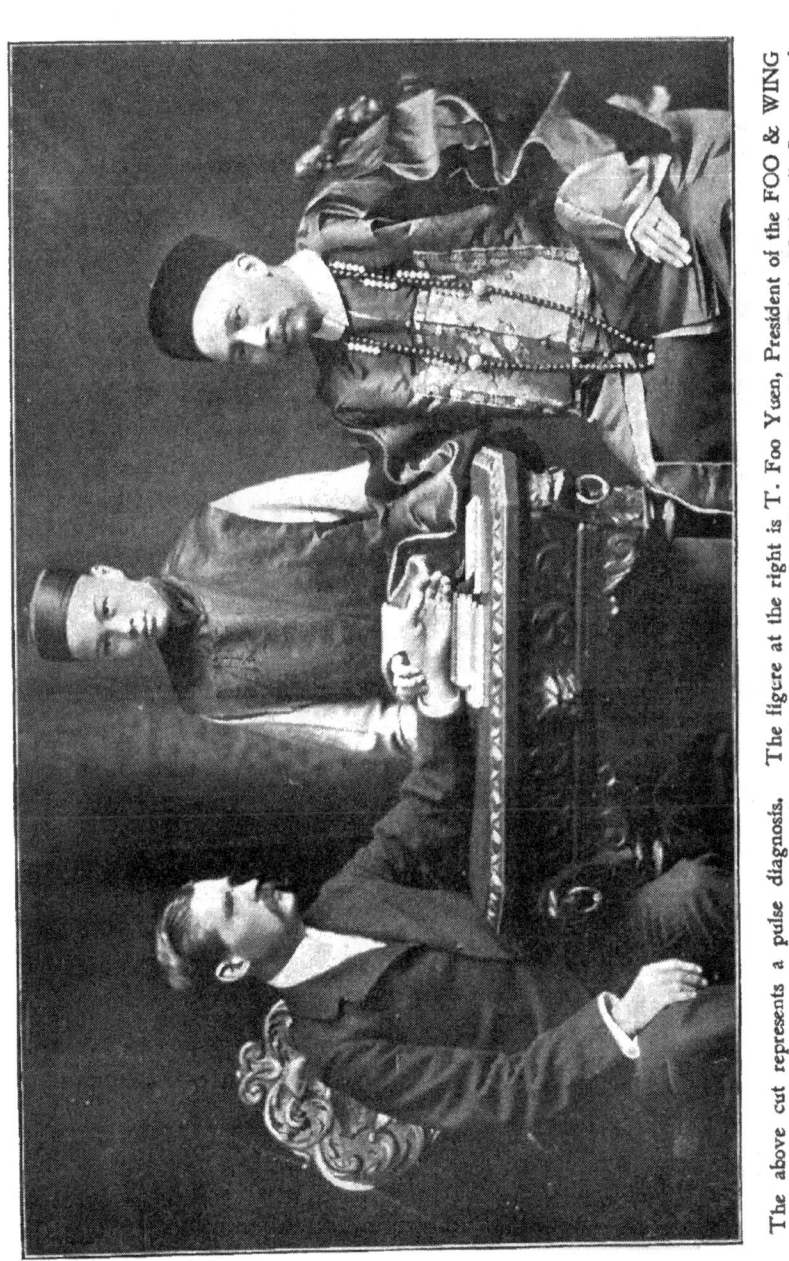

The above cut represents a pulse diagnosis. The figure at the right is T. Foo Yuen, President of the FOO & WING HERB COMPANY, that in the center is his son, Tom How Wing, the figure at the left is W. A. Hallowell, Jr., one of the friends of this corporation.

TREATISE NO. SIX **INVALUABLE TO INVALIDS**

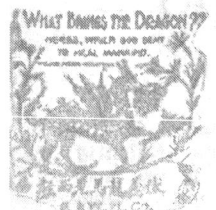

COMPLIMENTS OF
FOO & WING HERB CO.
903 S. Olive St. Los Angeles, C.

THE SCIENCE OF

ORIENTAL MEDICINE

ITS PRINCIPLES AND METHODS

COMPRISING

BIOGRAPHICAL SKETCHES OF ITS LEADING PRACTITIONERS, ITS TREATMENT OF VARIOUS PREVALENT DISEASES, USEFUL INFORMATION ON MATTERS OF DIET, EXERCISE AND HYGIENE . . . .

A GUIDE TO HEALTH

[Los Angeles]

COMPILED BY THE FOO & WING HERB COMPANY

INCORPORATED

Copyright 1902, by W. A. HALLOWELL, Jr.

TABLE OF CONTENTS.

CHAPTER I—Introductory information....A brief explanation of the principles and methods of the Oriental system of medicine.... The use of non-poisonous herbal remedies....Diagnosis by the pulse....Some comparisons with other systems. Pages 7 to 20.

CHAPTER II—Instruction on diet and hygiene....Bills of fare recommended....Special rules of diet for certain diseases....Diet in health....How the body derives sustenance from food....Directions for cooking....Valuable recipes for the preparation of food for invalids. Pages 20 to 72.

CHAPTER III—Information for patrons and inquirers....Suggestions on securing and preserving health....Some handy remedies.... Easy but useful exercises. Pages 72 to 87.

CHAPTER IV—Tom Foo Yuen, President of the Foo and Wing Herb Company....His diplomas and other credentials....A brief biographical sketch....His career in Southern California....Testimonials from patrons and friends....His plan for a college of Oriental medicine in America. Pages 87 to 113.

CHAPTER V—Tom Leong, vice-president of the Foo & Wing Herb Company....A brief sketch of his life and education. Pages 113 to 121.

CHAPTER VI—Some topics of Oriental medicine....Anatomy from the Chinese point of view....The medical profession in China ....The herbal remedies....Vivisection among the Chinese. Pages 121 to 150.

CHAPTER VII—The diseases of women....Testimonials. Pages 150 to 168.

CHAPTER VIII—Treatment of colds, malaria and paralysis....Testimonials. Pages 168 to 190.

CHAPTER IX—Treatment of asthma, consumption and hemorrhages ....Testimonials. Pages 190 to 208.

CHAPTER X—Treatment of cancers, abscesses, eczema, catarrh, bronchitis, rheumatism, neuralgia and heart troubles....Testimonials....A concise discussion of Oriental medicine. Pages 208 to 246.

CHAPTER XI—Treatment of piles or hemorrhoids, diphtheria, throat troubles, injuries to bones and cases usually supposed to require surgical treatment....Testimonials. Pages 246 to 263.

CHAPTER XII—Diseases of the eye....Cure of the liquor habit.... Appendicitis, its causes and cure. Pages 263 to 296.

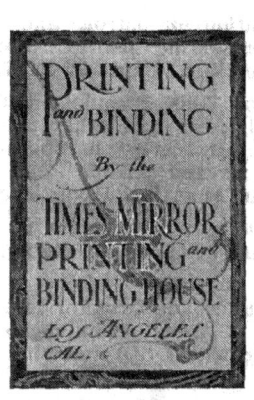

INTRODUCTION.

This book is offered to the public in the belief that it discusses matters of general interest and of vital importance to every family that it may reach. The subject of health is always interesting, and is uppermost in the thoughts of many people. Those who are not invalids will find in these pages several articles which are valuable as the productions of an educated Chinaman, and contain suggestions in reference to health and the care of the body which are worth while for any one to consider and to remember. The old adage that an ounce of prevention is worth a pound of cure applies to no other phase of human existence so fittingly as to the preservation of mental and bodily vigor. There are suggestions here which, if followed, may save years of suffering and regret.

Unfortunately, the great majority of the American people have already realized in their own experience, when too late, that it is much easier to keep health than to regain it when once lost. Our ways of life, filled with the excitements of pleasure, of society and of money-getting, bring the bitter with the sweet, and we have to pay for our nineteenth-century enjoyments not only in the coin of the realm, but in a thousand pains and aches through which nature takes revenge for the innumerable small violations of her laws. She has a summary way of inflicting her penalties in every case, that would teach the world better things were it not for the regretable, but undeniable, fact that nobody learns anything except through personal experience, which usually comes too late.

Recovery of lost health is an uphill struggle, and the worst feature of it is that the means usually employed are things that we so thoroughly dislike, bitter, nauseous doses, that we would be afraid to take in health, but are compelled to swallow in sickness, when one would naturally suppose that they would do us the most harm. It is an odd thing, if you will stop to think of it, that, just as soon as a man is taken ill, he is compelled, or at least advised, to take into his stomach some substance dug out of a mine or distilled from a poisonous plant. This does not seem rational, but it is the established custom.

The Chinese never fell into this way of medical practice. For centuries the use of all minerals and of all poisonous herbs or other substances has been forbidden by law in the Flowery Kingdom, and, with the off-hand ways of trial and punishment in vogue in that country, it would have been all a man's life was worth to prescribe opium, arsenic or any similar substance. The result is that a system of medicine has been practised in China for centuries which depends for its results solely upon strictly non-poisonous substances. In the opinion of the writer, the marvelous results attained by this system of medicine is due largely to this fact, and perhaps also to the peculiar method of diagnosis employed, through which the physician judges of the patient's condition through the pulse alone. The delicacy of touch and the quickness of perception attained by experts in this system is something simply marvelous and can be appreciated only by a personal experience.

Some of the following articles have been printed in the newspapers of Los Angeles and are here presented in convenient form for preservation and reference. Those who desire to know more of this method of healing than is here presented are cordially invited to call at the office of the Foo and Wing Herb Company, at No. 903 South Olive, this city, for a free consultation, diagnosis by the pulse, and opinion. You will find ladies and gentlemen of your own race in attendance and ready to offer every assistance. There is nothing hidden about this company, but the fullest investigation is cordially invited.

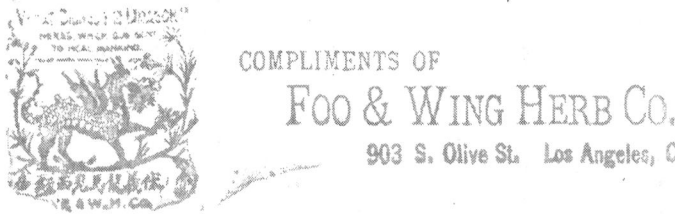

COMPLIMENTS OF
FOO & WING HERB CO.
903 S. Olive St. Los Angeles, Cal.

CHAPTER I.

INTRODUCTORY INFORMATION.

Some Facts About the Oriental System of Medicine—Its History and Principles.

For the benefit of those who do not understand the principles underlying the true Oriental system of medicine, as practiced in China, its use of herbal remedies and its theories of disease and anatomy, its method of diagnosis, its treatment and care of patients, we shall offer a brief discussion of the principles upon which this system is based, and shall tell something of its history and the reasons for its existence and adoption by the great Chinese nation. Some of the earliest mentions of Chinese medicine are found in an article upon China contained in the revised edition of the Encyclopedia Britannica, an authority which no one will dispute, from which we quote as follows:

"The spacious seat of ancient civilization which we call China has loomed always so large to western eyes, and has, in spite of the distance, subtended so large an angle of vision that, at eras far apart, we find it to have been distinguished by different appellations, according as it was reached by the southern sea route or by the northern land route, traversing the longitude of Asia. In the former aspect, the name has nearly always been some form of the name Sin, Chin, Sina, China. In the latter point of view, the region in question was known to the ancients as the land of Seres; to the middle ages as the Empire of Cathey. (Page 1539).

"Cathey is the name by which the Chinese Empire was known to mediaeval Europe, and is in its original form (Kitai) that by which China is still known in Russia and to most of the nations of Central Asia. (Page 1540).

"The notice of Rubruk runs thus: 'Further on is great Cathey, which I take to be the country which was anciently called the Land of the Seres, for the best silk stuffs are still got from them. The sea lies between it and India. Those Cathayans are little fellows, speaking much through the nose, as in general with all those Eastern people, their eyes are very narrow. They are first-rate artists in every kind of manufacture, and their physicians have a thorough knowledge of the virtue of herbs, and an admirable skill in diagnosing by the pulse.'"

Now Rubruk, quoted above by the Encyclopedia Britannica, was a celebrated traveler of the twelfth century. The evidence is undisputed, and it necessarily follows that in the twelfth century, the Chinese were practicing their herbal system of medicine, were diagnosing diseases by their pulse diagnosis, a method entirely distinct from that practiced in Europe at that time or since, and were very skillful in the treatment of disease. It is needless to ask what was the state of medicine in Europe at that time. All students of history are aware that it was in a very primitive and barbarous condition. The Chinese, therefore, had their system perfected and in successful operation long before there were doctors in Europe worthy of the name, and centuries before the discovery of America.

Such was the report of Chinese civilization and particularly of Chinese medicine brought back by Rubruk, the daring adventurer and explorer who had ventured into strange and unknown lands. But Chinese civilization was old when Rubruk saw it—centuries old, and Chinese medicine was as old as Chinese civilization. In fact, this system was spread throughout Asia at least 3000 years ago. Hence it was more than 2000 years old when Rubruk saw it and recorded the results of his observations, and the peculiar thing about it is that it has been consistent and unchanging from the beginning.

When the Chinese commenced to study medicine they went at once to the root of the different questions involved by practicing vivisection. Thousands of condemned criminals were taken and cut to pieces for the benefit of the living. In this way the functions of the vital organs, such as the kidneys, the liver, the stomach, the spleen and the heart were studied in the living person. The intensely important questions involved in the digestion of foods were determined as well as the effects of different drugs. These investigations, made while the man was still alive, were a thousand times more thorough and reliable than the guesswork which civilized physicians have practiced for many years by cutting up the bodies of dead men, when heat, motion and life are gone, and death has destroyed every function Another important point established in this way was that the pulsations at three different points on each wrist show the condition of the vital organs of the human body, a fact which is the basis of the pulse method of diagnosis. According to our ideas vivisection is very cruel, but .. is not necessary for us to discuss this phase of the subject except to say that 3000 years ago human life in any part of the world was held much cheaper than it is today in America. It may be questioned, moreover, whether vivisection was any more cruel than the methods of execution in vogue not so many hundred years ago in England, when men were hanged, drawn and quartered, burned at the stake, and put to death in many other cruel ways.

The benefits of the practice, from a medical point of view, cannot be denied. In fact, high medical authorities in this country and in Europe have earnestly advocated its practice, within recent years One of these men is Professor Pyle, of the medical college at Canton, Ohio, who recently presented a bill before the legislature of that state permitting the vivisection of criminals condemned to death for the benefits of science and humanity. Dr. Pyle, in his argument in support of this bill, proposed to do exactly what the Chinese did centuries ago. He stated that he would expose the stomach of the condemned and study the action of foods and liquids and of drugs. In this way definite results would be reached, and we would understand exactly many processes which, like the growing of a blade of grass, are matters of every day experience, yet are hidden deep beyond the limit of human understanding. In fact, this is acknowledged to be the only way of arriving at a correct knowledge of these subjects, the importance of which is perhaps greater than that of any others which concern the human race. But it is needless to say that no legislature has ever granted permission to vivisect criminals, and it is doubtful whether any legislature ever will. Americans know nothing of the action of the medicines which they take into their stomachs except by final effects. They can tell what the medicines do, but not how they do it, and they are ignorant whether the process, in many cases, as a whole, is a benefit or an injury Consequently everybody distrusts medicine and doctors, although compelled by the greater fear of death to take medicines and to employ doctors.

The Chinese, having made thorough investigations by means of vivisection, laid down the law at the start that no poisonous drugs whatever, and no minerals should be employed in the practice of medicine. This law has ever since been rigidly enforced. Invariable respect for this principle has prevailed, and no authenticated Chinese physician would think of prescribing opium, mercury or any similar substance. Through centuries of teaching the common people have also been educated to a horror of these so-called medicinal substances. And the result is that they are not used at all in Chinese medicine.

The theory of Chinese medicine, in general, is that a substance which can be used for food is suitable for use as medicine, and that a substance which would be poisonous or otherwise injurious as food is not only useless as medicine, but actually hurtful. The Chinese believe that one has no right to force upon a sickly, perhaps broken-down constitution, substances which would injure sound constitutions. Alcohol is a poison which they never use in the preparation of their remedies. They strive to strengthen and build up by the use of vegetable substances, many of which are really foods in special form, which are readily absorbed into the system, make new and rich blood, and through the blood nourish and sustain the body, just as any form of wholesome food nourishes and sustains. No one can allege this fact of morphine, strychnine, arsenic, nux-vomica, belladona, aconite, digitalis and a thousand and one other medicines which are prescribed every day by American physicians.

Again, the Chinese do not believe in using concentrated medicinal elements in the sense that American physicians employ them. It is the habit of the latter and of all manufacturers of medicinal preparations, in order to disguise the taste of the materials employed, to present them in as concentrated a form as possible. Therefore, a little very powerful medicine is taken into the system which is expected to do a great deal of work. The Chinese avoid this extreme. They do not attempt to accomplish results so quickly or so easily or with so little shock to the sense of taste. Everybody takes every day a great deal of food into the stomach in order to assimilate a comparatively small portion of it, which sustains us from day to day. After the same analogy the Chinese give larger doses of less concentrated medicines, and almost always in liquid form. This is absorbed into the system, and, without violent action, but gradually and surely it accomplishes the desired result. The longest way around is often the surest way home, and cures are frequently accomplished in a few days or weeks by these simple, harmless, vegetable substances which have resisted all the efforts of modern medical science for months and even years.

These facts are not stated to antagonize American physicians or to decry their methods of practice. The Oriental Herbal System of Medicine is so entirely different from any system in common use in America that there can be no comparison between them as to their respective merits, and these references to the methods of other physicians are made simply to illustrate our meaning and not with the intention of adverse criticism. The world is wide, and there is room for all. We do not wish to be insolent toward others or unnecessarily incur resentment and arouse bitterness. The facts speak for themselves. The Oriental system has cured thousands of cases of various forms of disease which had been abandoned by other doctors. This has been established beyond the possibility of dispute. In fact, we prefer to treat so-called incurable cases. As a rule Caucasians have been unwilling to consult us until they had tried every other form of medical treatment within their reach. Therefore, it may be said that all of the cures which we have made have been of cases given up by other doctors. We have hundreds of testimonials for these cures, and there are hundreds of people in Southern California who are now outspoken in upholding our system of medicale treatment, and make no secret of the fact that they have been cured by us, have confidence in us, and employ our methods whenever they believe themselves in need of medical attention. In other words, we have lived in Southern California long enough to establish a reputation, and to secure a following. This being true, we claim a right to recognition, and to state our principles and to explain our methods of practice, without malice toward any others.

We are firm believers in preventive medicine, in teaching correct living and in checking the progress of disease before it has reached a stage to be dangerous to life or incurable. To arrest the progress of a disease in its early stage is far better than to cure it when it has become chronic, because a great deal of suffering is saved and the result is much more certain. Fewer chances are taken because the patient's vitality is not so much impaired and there is more to build upon. Most people today are so afraid of doctors that they do not seek medical advice at the first symptom of disease, as they ought to do. They let the trouble run along because they do not want to be dosed with poisonous substances, and the result is that, after a little, there is need for ten times the amount of dosing that would have been required in the first place. If these same people knew that they could be treated by harmless vegetable substances, roots, herbs, barks, berries and flowers similar in their nature to substances which are eaten every day, medicines which do not derange the stomach or establish, like the morphine habit, greater difficulties than they are intended to cure, then they would take treatment at the outset when everything is in favor of recovery, instead of waiting until all the chances are against recovery; and the percentage of cures as compared to the number of invalids would take a sudden rise. There is something wrong in establishing methods in this respect. There are more doctors than can find practice, and each year brings forth a multitude of new discoveries in practice and in remedies. Yet the army of invalids constantly grows larger, showing that the discoveries, the remedies and the doctors do not accomplish what they undertake. In our opinion there are two principal reasons for this deplorable condition of affairs. One is that the people are not educated to the value of preventive medicine; the other is that American physicians have no correct theories of the origin and basis of life, and a very imperfect understanding of the correct functions and exact workings of the twelve vital organs.

Now, as to the position of the Chinese upon these two important points: In regard to the first, the whole Chinese nation is fully educated as to the value of preventive medicine. So true is this that the better class among the Chinese take regular courses of medicine, once or twice a year, for the purpose of purifying the blood, correcting the digestive powers and toning up the system in general. The result is that they avoid many attacks of sickness, and the Chinese nation, as a whole, is a remarkably healthy people. Even the poorest understand that, at the first symptoms of disease, they must use great care in diet, and some of the simple remedies with which all are familiar. A doctor's advice in China does not cost much, where every physician of repute sees from two hundred to three hundred patients a day. Moreover, the Chinese are not afraid of the remedies employed. They know that these will not harm them under any circumstances, and will probably do them good. They take medicine and regulate their diet and manners of life so as to keep well, and the result is that they are less often exposed to the perils of critical illness than the people of other countries. And many of the contagious diseases so prevalent in Europe and America, as consumption, for example, are practically unknown in China.

In reference to the second point, we have already explained that vivisection gave the Chinese at the outset definite ideas and facts concerning the normal functions of the vital organs, facts which cannot be determined from any number of examinations of those organs after death, when their very substance is impaired by disease and the vitalizing principle which keeps them in healthful action has departed forever from the body. The nations of Europe and America have never had the benefit of such observations upon the living and healthy subject. Hence we have the spectacle of thousands of learned men devoting their lives to building an elaborate and costly system of medicine, upon the truth of which the lives and health of millions of people depend, upon a foundation which is intact, incomplete and largely the merest guesswork. That science which should be the most certain of all sciences is admittedly the most wavering and the most changeable. Physicians are constantly abandoning established theories and taking up with whatever is new and untried, and perhaps, better than the old. Consequently medicine with the Caucasian is a succession of experiments, while the Chinese are still curing disease by the methods and the remedies which have been tested for centuries.

Take the spleen for instance. American physicians do not hesitate to admit their ignorance of its action and functions. In fact, they are inclined to poke fun at anyone who claims to know, and regard him as either an imposter or an ignoramus. Yet it is evident that the spleen must have been put into the human body for some useful purpose, and the Chinese know what that purpose is. They know that it is a very important factor in the processes of digestion, and they know just how it assists in those processes They know what remedies will assist it; something that the American doctor cannot know if he does not know what the organ is for. The Chinese have definite theories of anatomy in reference to every organ, and their philosophy goes deeper into many questions than that of any other nation. Here, again, vivisection set them right on the start, and they have never abandoned the facts which they discovered in this way.

The Oriental method of diagnosis is by the pulse alone, three fingers being used upon each wrist. By this method of examination is determined the condition of each vital organ, the derangement of any one, or of all of them, as the case may be, and the seat of the disease. No other examination is ever made except in case of external injury. This doubtless seems mysterious and impossible to many people, but their doubts can easily be removed if they will make a personal test of the matter. Only from three to five minutes time is required for an expert by this method to inform the person under examination of his good or ill health, his weakness or strength, and, sometimes, of the location of the various pains and aches which have disturbed him. Nearly everyone who has ever submitted to an examination by the pulse has been greatly surprised by its results. We ask no questions except, sometimes, the age of the person, and whether married or single. We sometimes also look at the patient's tongue. No charge is ever made for examination and diagnosis. Patients are always instructed upon the correct theory of diet and ways of life, and, although our ideas upon these subjects are new to the people of the United States, yet nearly everyone who becomes familiar with them at once recognizes their value. They appeal to common sense and to universal experience. And all have agreed that our theory of diet is far in advance of any other taught upon this continent.

The Oriental remedies are usually administered in the form of herb teas. These teas are made from herbs indigenous to Asia, which are gathered on the mountains and in the valleys of China, and are imported directly by ourselves. More than 3000 different species of these herbs are in use, comprising roots, barks, flowers, leaves and berries. From ten to eighteen kinds of these herbs are used in each prescription. From two to six cups of water are added and then boiled down to one cup, which is a dose for an adult, and is drunk hot. The dose is varied to suit the strength and constitutional power or vitality of the patient, as determined by pulse examination Changes in these are at once apparent in the pulse, and the effect of each dose is ascertained before another is administered This is important, because medicines have different effects upon people of different constitutional powers. In serious cases a daily examination is made as long as the patient is under treatment, but in less severe cases, after the strength of the medicine to be prescribed has once been decided, less frequent examinations, say every other day, or once in three days, are sometimes sufficient It is sometimes necessary to give a test treatment of a week or ten days to ascertain the effect the remedies will have in a given case before we can decide whether the case is curable or not. Many cases apparently hopeless have been restored to health. One dose of medicine, that is, a full cup of tea, a day is the usual rule. But sometimes two doses a day are given, and sometimes the one cup is divided into two doses and given at shorter or longer intervals, according to circumstances.

Nearly all of the prescriptions are varied often. It is rare that one runs for more than five days without some change in proportion, or by leaving out one ingredient or more, and substituting others. This is true even of chronic cases which require treatment from three to fifteen months. The herb teas are always to be taken on an empty stomach. Sometimes in the early morning, between two o'clock and five, sometimes an hour or so before breakfast, dinner or supper, or at bedtime, but always from three and a half to four hours after a meal. The intention is to have the stomach empty of foods so that there may be nothing to interfere with the action of the remedies, and also so that the stomach may be prepared for the next meal by that action. We explain all forms of food, meats, fruits, vegetables, drinks, cereals, etc , and show which are beneficial and which are injurious to our patients while taking our remedies. We consider the diet that we prescribe to be fully as essential as the remedies, and we insist upon our patrons observing our bills of fare. We show them that the success of the treatment depends upon this. Medicine is of no value whatever if the food taken counteracts it, but the food and the medicine should work together. Then the patient gets the full nutritive value of the food which he eats, and his recovery is hastened rather than retarded.

After all, success is the true test of the merit of any system, and by this standard we are prepared to compare ours with any other. The results show that we have a thorough knowledge of the Chinese system of medicine and theory of life, which are founded upon a complete understanding of Nature's laws. Americans carry their theories of science to extremes and get too far away from the simple, fundamental facts upon which health depends. The hardest cases we find to cure are those who have been the rounds of the scientific men, sometimes traveling from one end of the continent to the other, testing every conceivable form of medication, often including mineral waters at so-called health resorts, and hundreds of patent medicines. The substances in these agencies misnamed medicinal, permeate the whole body, accumulate in the pores of the skin, the muscles and tissues, and the very substance of the bones itself. All of these poisons have to be dislodged before recovery is possible. Nine-tenths of the chronic sufferers from disease are poisoned through and through as a result either of their own ignorance and neglect of Nature's laws or of unsuccessful attempts to cure them after they had begun to lose their health. To take these people and rescue them not only from the grasp of disease, but also from the additional burdens of unsuccessful medication is certainly a test of the highest skill. But we have accomplished it over and over again, and the results have often seemed miraculous to those who have witnessed them in only a few instances. After they have seen the same results accomplished repeatedly they begin to understand that knowledge, not magic, works wonders

In these difficult cases from three to four months' time is required to effect a change in the blood, without which recovery is impossible. This is what we call a course of medicine. Usually one course is sufficient for a cure, but in obstinate cases two, three or even four or five courses may be necessary to reinstate the patient's health. This depends, of course, entirely upon the patient's condition, the extent of the ravages of the disease, whatever it may be, upon the vital organs and the constitutional power. Age also has much to do with the length of time required for a cure. The teas almost always agree with even the weakest stomachs. Children and even infants take them without hesitation after the first dose or two, and the stomach very rarely rejects them. They leave no disagreeable taste in the mouth, and these facts show that they are in harmony with the human body and its functions.

Our treatment is always thorough and persistent. We expect that patients will co-operate in every possible way by following directions implicitly, even when they involve a certain degree of self sacrifice. We hold that considerations of health are infinitely higher than any possible consideration of pleasure or convenience, and that, when a man is in pursuit of lost health, everything else should take second place, if necessary. Our patrons soon see the reasonableness of this position, and the fact that we are firm with them gives them all the greater confidence in us. It is absurd, when fighting disease, to fight also improper food, irregular hours and dissipation of various kinds. Instead of these disadvantages the patient should have the assistance of a correct, wholesome and nutritious diet, regularity in eating, exercise and rest, and avoidance of all undue excitement or excess. Better have all possible elements of the problem of health on your side than to array them all against you and then depend upon medicine alone to do the work. The latter course is to invite failure, which we do not propose to do, for we fully realize our responsibility when we examine a patient and undertake to cure him.

Surgery in China is a distinct profession from that of medicine, and we never resort to the use of the knife, but we do accomplish through medicines alone, taken internally or applied externally, many things which are commonly supposed to be impossible. Our treatment avoids many painful, uncertain and risky surgical operations, which are too often a last resort after medication has failed. If medication were more often successful there would be little surgery necessary. We have shown many times that our herbal remedies cure many diseases, the diseases of women for instance, which have been too often treated by surgical interference as a last resort, after physicians and "specialists" had tried in vain to cure them by medication. The difference is that our remedies nourish and repair the organs of the human body in addition to their medicinal effect. Whenever surgery conflicts with medicine there is a confession that the latter is a failure, for surgery never cures. It is simply a last resort, to make the patient as well as possible under the circumstances, and to prevent greater injury than has already been done by cutting away the seat of disease, not by curing the disease.

We have often been asked: "What is your specialty?" We reply that we treat all derangements of the human system, but are not so particular as some other physicians in naming them. We ascertain what organs are diseased and the extent of the injury, and we apply the remedies which help those organs to throw off the disease or to recover from the derangement. If more than one organ is involved we treat all that are involved. The normal and harmonious performance of the functions of all the vital organs is health. The derangement of one or more is disease. This is the whole question in a nutshell. Names are a very minor consideration Naming a disease does not help to cure it nor to preserve life. A hundred persons may be in ill health, with different symptoms of disease, yet the cause of the trouble in each may be substantially the same. It would be illogical to treat the outward symptoms in these cases. The true way is to prescribe for the organ or organs involved. Then the outward symptoms, in all their varied forms, disappear and the cure is established. If a tree is dying for want of water the best way is to apply water to the roots, and the beneficial effect will be felt everywhere from the roots to the leaves. It is the same with the human body. If the vital organs can be kept normal in their action these take care of the rest of the body and there is no unpleasant symptoms of disease except from external injuries.

As a general rule, in the case of a confirmed invalid, there can be no permanent cure without a thorough cleansing of the system. When the processes of digestion and elimination have been deranged for some time there are certain to be impurities in the system which clog the blood, obstruct all the functions and even penetrate the tissues and the very marrow of the bones. The longer the case has gone without help the worse is this condition. It is useless, under these circumstances, to attempt a cure by outward applications of plasters, poultices, inhalations or injections, or to attempt to build up a weakened system by so-called strengthening foods, which it cannot assimilate and use. The source of the disease still remains as active as ever in spite of these palliative measures, which are usually absolutely ineffective. The system must first be cleansed. Then the vital organs can do their work properly and without hindrance. If the digestive organs and juices are first restored to a normal condition digestion becomes again perfect and the patient thrives and gains flesh and strength on ordinary foods, and even on those that are usually considered very plain and light foods, without an attempted forcing upon the system of heavy, oily substances, which are distasteful to a strong stomach, and cannot possibly be taken up by a weak one. There is no use in adding fuel to a fire that is covered and clogged with ashes. Rake away the encumbering mass first, then apply your fuel and a blaze is the result; but if the spark hidden in dead material cannot be reached because of that material it cannot be made to burn into a flame. So the weakened human body will resume its normal functions when the impurities are taken out of its way, and not before.

But before anything whatever can be accomplished a correct diagnosis is indispensable. In very many cases this can only be obtained by the pulse method. Hundreds of patients have told us that ours was the first and only correct diagnosis they had ever had in their cases. We cannot dwell here upon the reasons for our expertness in this direction, except to say that an inherited gift has been cultivated to the highest degree of efficiency by long and patient practice. There are many examples of equal expertness in other branches of human endeavor which illustrate this. The blind, for instance, cultivate the sense of touch until it takes the place of the sense of sight to a great extent. The musician cultivates the sense of hearing until he can detect the slightest discordant note in the loud burst of an orchestral music. A discord which is absolutely unnoticed by the ordinary ear. So long practice has enabled us to detect the minute signs of distress and decay which the vital organs send to the wrist through the medium of the pulse. When the source of the difficulty is thus absolutely defined, the proper remedies can be prescribed with a reasonable certainty of benefit in every case, and the chances of failure are reduced to the lowest.

CHAPTER II.

OUR BILLS OF FARE.

VALUABLE RECIPES FOR INVALIDS.

Some Rules in Reference to Diet, Exercise and Hygiene.

We are very particular about the diet of our patrons. The general rule in this regard is to avoid all foods which are too strong and tend to produce inflammation, and all foods which contain little or no nutriment and therefore impose a useless burden upon the digestive powers; also all foods which are made up principally of sweets and acids, because these are likely to ferment in the stomach and are of no value as nourishment It should be remembered in this connection that persons taking these medicines require much less food than others.

For purposes of convenience in reference we divide our list of foods into three bills of fare. No. 1 is for weak people or those in a somewhat advanced stage of disease, or those who are taking strong medicines. It is very important that these persons should not overload the stomach.

BILL OF FARE NO. 1.

Mushes and Cereals.

Steamed or Boiled Rice.   Rolled Oats.   Rolled Wheat.   Corn Meal.
Wheatena.   Graham Mush.   Germea.   Farina.
Wheat Grits.

Soups.

All Vegetable Soups.
Soups prepared with Macaroni and Vermicelli.
Cream of Celery Soup and other soups prepared with Milk.
Gruels made of Rice, Barley or Oatmeal.

Meat and Eggs.

Beef Stew.   Young Duck.   Young Beef or Veal.
The whites of two eggs, prepared as directed under the heading "To Cook Eggs," or a Poached Egg or Egg Timbales, according to the recipes given below.

Vegetables.

Boiled Green Peas.   Young Mustard.   Lettuce, Greens or Spinach.
Lentils and Split Peas.   Steamed, Baked or Boiled Potatoes, either Sweet or Irish.

Bread.

Meek's Aerated Bread, either White, Graham or Whole Wheat.
Gems made from Gluten or Whole-Wheat Flour.
Corn Bread.   Boston Brown Bread.   Shredded Wheat Biscuit.
Graham and other Crackers and Hard Biscuits.
White Bread a little Stale.
Toast, either Dry, Buttered, Cream or Milk.

Butter may be used, but not to excess. Patients on this bill of fare should be careful in this respect.

Desserts.

Very plain Puddings made from Rice, Sago, Tapioca or Farina.
Custards.   A little Grape, Currant or Guava Jelly.
Fig or Blackberry Jam.   Unfermented Grape Juice.

Fruits.

Patients whose health is delicate should be careful in the use of fruits while taking our remedies. Cooked fruits are always better than raw. Those whose digestion is impaired or whose condition, for any reason is serious, should use no raw fruits whatever. They may eat cooked pears, apples, figs, blackberries and prunes.

Drinks.

With this bill of fare we recommend only boiled water, boiled milk, weak black tea and perhaps a little cocoa or chocolate. We shall discuss the question of drinks and thirst more fully in a later paragraph.

Sufficient Nourishment Given.

We consider that this bill of fare will afford ample nourishment for delicate persons. The cereals, boiled milk and a little meat should be the foundation of the diet, other articles being added for variety.

All meats must be used with caution if there is any fever. If there is no fever then meats may be used more freely. Milk is excellent food for all who can use it. It may be used by our patrons in all cases where there is no coughing or raising of phlegm, but if either of these is present milk should be employed only sparingly. A little cream may be given on mushes, cereals, puddings, toast or baked apples.

BILL OF FARE NO. 2.

When patients are stronger and their digestion is better, and there is little or no fever, the following foods may be added to those mentioned above:

Turkey, squirrel, venison, chocolate and cocoa may be used more freely than in bill of fare No. 1 Coffee is forbidden. Birds are too strong for invalids. Soups and broths made from lean meat and prepared after some of the receipts given below may be used. White lima or string beans, asparagus, cooked celery and ripe olives may be added to bill of fare No. 1.

BILL OF FARE NO. 3.

When our patrons are still better they may add certain foods to the bill of fare No. 2. Young chicken may be used. The pullets are preferable as the meat is less strong and less likely to cause inflammation. A small amount of boiled ham may be employed, also some lamb. Lamb is good for strengthening the system, but should not be eaten if the patient has any poison or eczema in his system. This meat is too strong for an impure system. A little broiled bacon may be used, well done. Patients may now also eat all kinds of fish, except oysters, crabs, lobster and other shell fish, which are not good at any time. Lobsters and crabs are more injurious than oysters. They may use water cress, green corn, turnips, lima and white beans.

NOTE.

In many diseases where the person is suffering from nerve exhaustion or other weakness, and where there is no fever and the digestive organs are not seriously impaired, the person need not commence with bill of fare No. 1 and proceed gradually to the others, but may select his articles of diet from any of the foods permitted in either of the bills of fare. But in acute cases, especially where there is fever, the bills of fare must be strictly followed. In all cases the articles forbidden must be avoided. And the special directions for diet for the different diseases must also be followed. When all fever is gone and the person improves, greater freedom in diet may be permitted except as regards those articles absolutely prohibited.

GENERAL SUGGESTIONS ON DIET.

All fruits should be cooked. Then the acid digests easily. But in cases when there is diarrhoea or indigestion, or a raising of mucus or phlegm, the use even of cooked fruits should be less. In some of these cases a very little fruit may be used, but great caution must be observed. Sometimes dried fruits, such as dried pears, raisins and figs are better than any other fruits, because they contain less acid, and they are therefore better in the above kinds of sickness. But all fruits allowed, whether dried or fresh, should be cooked. The patient and his friends must use judgment in all of these matters.

The following vegetables and fruits are not good and are to be avoided at all times: Tomatoes, squash, pumpkin, peaches, apricots, all kinds of plums, pine apples and muskmelons. Apricots and peaches are especially injurious in skin diseases and after attacks of measles.

Remember that nature is always kind to man as long as he obeys her commands. But if he persists in transgressing her laws then he must take the consequences. If ill health has been induced by an improper mode of life, the first thing to do is to get back as close to nature as is possible. In the matter of foods this means plain food and not too much of that. Improper food is the cause of most of the ills of life, and most of the diseases that afflict mankind. Use no concentrated foods, no foods heavy with starch or sugar, no lard or similar highly carbonaceous food, no finely bolted flour. As a rule the fruits of California have too much acid. If they are eaten freely they burn or dry up the gastric juices. Then comes thirst. There is a deficiency of gastric juices for the digestion of the food. When coffee is taken under these circumstances the situation is still worse. It adds to the dryness of the stomach and intestinal tract and brings on constipation, liver troubles and nervousness. One who has any stomach trouble, indigestion or gastric difficulties, should avoid everything cooked in hot air. All foods should be steamed or boiled.

Patrons of this system must necessarily use judgment in reference to all articles of diet not included in our bills of fare. We have given what we consider an ample variety for all persons suffering from any disease sufficiently severe to require a course of medication Still, some little latitude may be allowed in the choice of other foods. These bills of fare apply especially to the climate of Southern California, which is a warm climate. Persons living in a colder climate may, perhaps, use some more highly carbonaceous foods to advantage. In a general way, all sweets, acids, very cold foods or drinks, and all stimulants should be avoided, also raw fruits.

AS TO THINGS TO DRINK.

We have constant inquiries from persons who suffer from excessive thirst and desire permission to drink various things which are forbidden in our bills of fare. We think that we allow an ample variety when we permit hot or boiled water, hot milk, weak black tea, rice gruel, hot or cold lemonade, cocoa and chocolate. The cocoa and chocolate must be taken sparingly, for they are heavy, oily foods, and not easily digested. Remember that water alone will not quench thirst because it will not allay fever. The thirst from which many people suffer is not a natural condition. It indicates inward fever and a deficiency of gastric juices. The only way to cure it is to allay the inflammation and to grow up the gastric juices. This requires time. Our remedy No. 123 is the best thing known for this purpose, and the use of it for a few days or weeks will produce a remarkable change for the better. We have found hot water with a couple of teaspoonfuls of strained honey excellent. Water should always be filtered and boiled and taken hot. Those who work away from home and cannot get the water hot should boil it and take it with them and drink it cool But never take ice-cold drinks under any circumstances. They do not allay thirst at all, but simply add to the inflammation already existing. Ice-cold soda water and beer are the causes of innumerable derangements of the stomach. The fact that these are usually taken in the summer, when the weather is very hot, makes their use all the more detrimental, for the stomach is first heated by the hot breaths of summer and then suddenly cooled by the forced invasion of a quantity of ice-cold fluid, mixed with various syrups and gases which make it pleasant to the taste but destructive of health.

GOOD ADVICE FROM AN AMERICAN PHYSICIAN.

In this connection we desire to reprint the following from a recent article in the Los Angeles Times, written by an American physician, which contains much sound advice upon the subject of what people ought to drink. After some discussion of the evils of using alcoholic drinks the writer continues as follows:

"After all, however, straight whisky or brandy, if pure and taken in small quantities, is probably the least harmful of alcoholic beverages Beer, as it is consumed in this country, contains a large amount of carbonic acid gas, and then, it is always served far too cold to be wholesome. You will notice that a German usually warms his glass of beer with the hands before he consumes it. In Europe they would never dream of serving it at such a low temperature There is no question that the extensive consumption of iced beverages is one of the leading causes of dyspepsia in this country, and is also one of the causes of Bright's disease. In addition to these drawbacks all beer, except that which is made on the spot, contains salicylic acid, or some other preservative. The same drawbacks—carbonic acid gas and low temperature—apply to all the drinks sold at drug stores, in addition to which, some of these, such as cocoa and bromide beverages, which have become so popular during the past few years, possess dangerous qualities of their own.

Of the numerous liqueurs, chartreuse is probably the most wholesome. It has medicinal qualities, the main component being pure olive oil. This, however, cannot be regarded as a beverage.

The light wines of the country contain only a moderate percentage of alcohol, and are usually regarded as the most wholesome form of alcoholic beverage. This is doubtless true, but even here we are confronted by the fact that a great majority of the California wines contain salicylic acid. This caused one of our local dealers a considerable amount of trouble and loss some years ago, when he sent a shipment of California wine to Mexico, where the government appears to be more careful than ours of the health of its citizens. Sweet wines, such as port, sherry, angelica and muscatel, should be avoided by those who value their digestive organs, especially the sweet wines made in California. They are an artificial beverage, the fermentation being arrested by the addition of brandy, and will work havoc in the interior department of a human being quicker than any other variety of alcoholic beverage. A morning headache, following an indulgence in such wine, is something long to be remembered, even by a confirmed worshipper of Bacchus. Fruit juice, or "unfermented wine," is likely to recommence fermentation when it lies in the warm stomach.

Suppose we eliminate alcoholic beverages altogether, we are still far from an easy solution of the question what to drink. Tea, unless taken in limited quantities, and weak, will produce nervousness and other disorders in the average person. We have not, like the Chinese, been accustomed to the use of tea for hundreds, or even thousands of years. Coffee hardens and injures the liver, on account of which a number of substitutes have been placed on the market of late, and have met with a large sale. These usually consist of mixed grains, roasted and ground, and from a hygienic standpoint are certainly *...ocolate, as sold ... starch, which is not a very wholesome food. Again, these beverages cannot be readily assimilated by many stomachs. Milk is regarded by many as an ideal beverage, but it should really never be taken as a beverage, but as a food. Milk was intended for infants, not for grown persons. It should never be taken in conjunction with meat. The injunction of Moses against boiling the lamb in its mother's milk has a hygienic foundation, like most of the other Jewish laws that we find in the Bible. If milk is used by grown persons, it should be sipped very slowly, and taken preferably hot. Indeed, hot drinks are better than the cold beverages so popular in this country. The general use of hot drinks by the Chinese, and their avoidance of cold liquors, is doubtless one of the reasons for the astonishing vitality they display. Buttermilk is a wholesome beverage for those who can digest it. It contains an acid which is good for the liver and digestion. Here again, however, we are confronted by the fact that much of the buttermilk sold in the cities contains a preservative.

We find, therefore, that if we wish to fix upon a beverage that is absolutely wholesome, we shall have to confine ourselves to water—pure mountain spring water, or distilled water—at a cold, but not icy temperature. There are, however, many who will not consent to this. For these the most wholesome and least harmful liquid menu would, probably be, for breakfast, a cup of weak, black tea—preferable Ceylon or Assam, on account of cleanliness in preparation—or cereal coffee, and for lunch and dinner a little California Riesling or claret, diluted with about half as much pure water without ice. If a 'nightcap' is taken—although it would better be omitted—a glass of hot Scotch is about the best thing to take, although a cup of herb tea would do the stomach more good and tend to produce pleasanter dreams.

Again it should be repeated that alcohol is in no sense of the word a food, is not necessary, and is always more or less injurious, in whatever form it may be taken. If, however, a person believes, or imagines, that he must use alcoholic beverages, or simply desires to use them, whatever his belief may be, let him at least use judgment and not make a human hog of himself."

FOOD VALUE OF TEA.

There is much discussion among medical authorities in reference to the food value of tea. We are inclined to permit out patrons to use tea, to a reasonable extent, always with the proviso that it is to be taken weak by those in a weakened or serious condition, and never to excess by any. Tea is a stimulant and, especially when there is fever, it should be taken with caution. Nevertheless, it has a certain value as food. In this connection we quote the following paragraph which has been going the rounds of the press recently:

"FOOD VALUE OF TEA. We may state that one pound of good tea contains about a third of an ounce of theine, two and a half ounces of caseine, one-twelfth ounce of volatile oil, two and a half ounces of gum, half an ounce of sugar, half an ounce of fat, four ounces of tannic acid," says a noted American medical journal. Mineral matter of ash, water and woody fiber make up the remainder. Caseine, of which there is so large a quantity, it will be remembered, is the nutritive principle of milk; vegetable caseine, or legumen, is analogous in principle. Tea is, therefore, a highly nutritious substance, and fully capable of forming flesh and sustaining life. Peas and beans are highly concentrated forms of food, and yet analysis shows that the better qualities of tea are as rich in the nitrogenous element of nutriment principle as are these seeds. Caseine is identical in composition with the muscular fiber, and with the albumen of the blood, and is easy of assimilation."

COFFEE AND TOBACCO.

Tobacco burns out the juices of the system and injures the saliva upon which digestion largely depends. It is best for our patients to stop the use of tobacco entirely, if possible. If it is easy for you to drop off your cigars entirely you had better do so, but if this seems too hard, in the case of confirmed smokers, then you should smoke less, say one cigar in the morning and one in the evening, after dinner or supper. This measure of indulgence will not be enough to produce any great injury to the system. Our bill of fare is intended primarily for weak and sick people. After a cure is made it is, in many cases, better to follow the bill of fare, but this is not imperative. If you do not follow it for a time and see no bad effects from returning to your customary diet, then you can continue in that way and there will be no harm done. Everyone must decide this matter for himself, because what hurts one does not necessarily hurt another.

The same reasoning applies to coffee. After you are cured you can drink a little coffee; you can also use roast and fried meats in moderation, which may help the natural heat of the body. But you must be careful to avoid excess in all of these matters. You should also use boiled and steamed meats, which assist the gastric juices more and are easier to digest than fried and roast meats, but the latter hurt the natural heat, and for that reason are bad. A little might not hurt the gastric juices, but excess will give rise to inflammation. If, after a cure, you stop following the bill of fare and find afterwards that you do not feel well or that there is some difficulty of digestion or other trouble, then you should take it up again and follow the bill of fare all the time. This shows that you cannot eat whatever you like, and that you must live plainly; that there is too much fire in your system, if the natural juices are helped you will feel good; if the natural heat is helped you will feel bad. But not many people have this temperament, although it applies to some, who should be put on their guard in this particular.

USEFUL HINTS.

The herb tea should be taken fully one hour before meal time, or about three hours after a meal. Four hours after is better; must be two hours at least.

Undigested food ferments, generating a gas, which increases the poisonous gases already in the system, adding fuel to flame, poisons the system and counteracts the effects of the medicine.

Weak people cannot digest a meal as quickly as healthy persons, therefore great care should be exercised to avoid taking anything into the stomach before the previous meal has been completely digested. When foods and liquids are taken into the stomach before the previous meal has been completely digested, the process of digestion will be interrupted; then the food will sour and ferment and generate a gas that will enter the circulation, poisoning the blood, causing more or less distress to weakly people.

DIET IN CERTAIN DISEASES.

Realizing that the most difficult question in cases of sickness is what the patient may be permitted to eat we give below special instructions on diet in several of the more common forms of disease. We have attempted to adapt the ordinary foods permitted by American physicians to our form of treatment as far as possible. But there are certain points of difference which must be brought to the attention of persons using our remedies in order to prevent confusion in their minds between our rules of diet and those recognized by American physicians. Some of these are the following:

Use of Stimulants.—American physicians, both in acute and chronic disorders, very frequently employ foods and liquids that are highly stimulating in order to keep up the strength of the patient Thus they prescribe alcohol in its various forms, whisky, brandy, gin, rum, wines of many kinds, and malt liquors, such as beer, ale and porter. Now we do not say absolutely that a dose of wine or whisky may not be in rare instances of some benefit. Yet we do not permit the use of these articles either as medicine or food. We believe that all stimulants must be avoided. This is particularly true in cases of fever. Our effort is directed towards restoring a natural condition of the system, developing the gastric juices and reducing the fever. Alcohol, in any form, and stimulating foods work against this effort. We permit no beef juice, rich broths or highly concentrated foods in fevers. They add fuel to the flame. In acute attacks of all kinds the simpler the food taken the better. Then our remedies have an opportunity to accomplish their work without combating both the disease and the food taken into the system. There is far more danger of the patient taking too much food than there is of his taking too little.

Use of Heavy Foods.—The same principle applies in other wasting diseases, such as tuberculosis or consumption. There is no use in loading the stomach of the patient with fats, hot blood, cod liver oil and similar substances which he cannot digest. We direct our efforts to clearing his system of poisons and restoring the digestive juices and processes to something like a normal condition. Then the patient will take on more flesh with a comparatively small amount of food than he will with great quantities, little of which is digested and assimilated.

Use of Liquids.—We do not permit our patients to drink ice-cold liquids of any kind. These do not quench thirst but often add to the inflammation which causes the thirst. They may give a little temporary relief, but the final result is to increase the thirst instead of rendering it less. We prefer that our patients should take their liquids hot, including hot water. This is the best for the system in every way, and hot water, even in cases of fever, will quench the thirst much quicker than ice-water. But sometimes, if patients tire of the hot water, they may be permitted water that is cool, but not ice cold. Some physicians teach that sick people should take a great amount of liquid in the shape of various drinks. This is unnecessary, in our opinion. Only a moderate quantity of liquids should be taken. Weak tea may be used in the place of tea and coffee, when patients feel that they must have some warm drink besides water. Plain soda water or mineral waters, cool, but not cold, may be taken if persons are fond of them.

Use of Sugars and Acids.—We desire our patrons to avoid the use of sweets, because they ferment and become acids in the stomach, and the use of all acids. These create an injurious condition of the blood, which we try to counteract by the use of our herbs. But there is no use in trying to work the acids out of a person's system by means of medicine if that person is constantly adding more through the mouth. In many cases this is very important, and patients must abstain entirely from all sugars and acids of every kind, including acid fruits. In milder cases a moderate amount of sugar may be taken with the food.

Spices and Highly-Seasoned Foods.—For similar reasons we forbid all spices and highly-seasoned foods, except a little pepper and salt. Foods prepared with mustard and heavy oils are most difficult of digestion and become a burden to the digestive organs which they are not prepared to bear in cases of sickness.

Our bills of fare give all of the ordinary foods which sick persons ought to eat. After recovery a little more latitude may be allowed. We shall now discuss some of the foods that are to be used in special diseases, and commence with the foods that may be employed in that very large class of cases wherein there is fever.

DIET IN CASES OF FEVER.

In fever there is always a very rapid wasting of the tissues of the body, because the fever burns these up and, at the same time prevents the degree of digestion necessary to repair them. The food in fevers must therefore be nutritious, but of a sort that will not add fuel to the flame and make the fever worse, and also of a sort that is easily digested. Fever always means a severe sickness, and therefore the patient has little appetite or ability to take much nourishment, although it is important that he should be well nourished. For this reason—the lack of appetite and the difficulty of digestion—no solid food should be taken, but all the food should be in liquid form, or in the form of soft foods, and care should be taken that the patient does not take too much at a time, for if the stomach is overloaded a part of the food remains and decomposes and adds to the difficulties of the case.

Milk is one of the best foods that we have in cases of fever. It contains all the elements that are necessary to sustain life and repair waste of tissue. It is best to take it hot, or it may be made into broths, with a little rice or arrowroot. Milk should always be sipped, eaten slowly. If taken too rapidly it forms a mass in the stomach that is very hard to digest. In severe cases, milk is really about the only safe food there is.

In cases of more moderate severity and of shorter duration, more freedom may be allowed in the choice of foods. Although no solid foods should be given and all meats are forbidden, yet semi-solid food may be permitted, such as milk toast or cream toast, soft cooked eggs, cooked in the shell or prepared as directed below under the head of "Egg Timbales," thoroughly boiled oatmeal gruel, or rice or barley gruel, plain rice pudding. The gruels used, except the rice, must be strained through a fine strainer or a cheese cloth bag. They may be salted and flavored, if desired, with a little cinnamon or clove. Grape sugar may also be added. Beef tea may be added to these gruels, if entirely free from fat or grease, or beaten eggs may be used. Eggs eaten alone should be slowly cooked, as described in the paragraph headed: "Another Good Way to Cook Eggs." Rice gruel prepared as directed in this chapter is a splendid food in all cases of fever and may be given often. It is a food, is soothing to the stomach and also supplies liquid to quench the thirst.

In addition to the rice gruel, a little sour lemonade, either hot or cool, may be taken, or weak tea. But if there is severe indigestion in the stomach, the tea should not be given. Barley water may be used in place of the rice water, if preferred, and may be flavored with cinnamon or sweetened with grape sugar.

As the patient begins to recover, the use of food must be very sparing at first, but may be gradually increase. And these patients usually develop a very active appetite. Such articles as poached eggs on toast, egg-nog, beef tea taken hot, jellies, custards, cream of celery soup, cocoa, tapioca or rice puddings, buttered toast, baked sweet apples with cream, baked potatoes, may be given for a few days, say from one to two weeks, and after that, more solid food may gradually be added, such as meats, poultry and game

TYPHOID FEVER.

In this severe form of fever especial care must be taken with the diet because the intestines are affected by the fever and any form of solid food would be very likely to lacerate the intestinal walls. If taken in time, our remedies break up typhoid fever and prevent a long sickness. But if the malady is fully started before our remedies are taken it may run a month, or even five or six weeks, and care must still be taken with the food for a period of from two weeks to two months after the patient begins to recover.

Milk is the best possible food in typhoid fever. And enough should be taken to keep up the strength of the patient as far as possible. This quantity will vary anywhere between one and three quarts per day. Probably in most cases, three ounces of milk every two and a half hours would be sufficient.

Milk is best given boiled. It may be diluted with plain hot water or with rice water. A little cocoa may be added, sometimes, to disguise the taste, if the patient tires of the plain milk. Sometimes typhoid patients lose flesh very rapidly, and, in these cases, the milk diet must be varied. Soups made from farina, arrowroot or rice may be given, or a little beef or mutton broth, if entirely free from fat and grease, custards, egg-nog, or the whites of eggs beaten up with cream, or with a little sherry wine, or with milk and sherry Plenty of rice gruel should be taken, and plenty of hot water. The mouth should be washed out very frequently and always after taking milk. A piece of cotton may be used for this purpose, and the tongue should be scraped with a spoon handle or a piece of bent whalebone.

No solid food should be taken for several days after the fever has gone down. Then, at first, rice, tapicoa, vermicelli, cream toast should be given, maccaroni, soft-cooked eggs, and finally, chicken or mutton or beef broths, then some of the vegetables, such as baked potatoes or cooked celery, then a little beef, mutton, chicken or game.

SCARLET FEVER AND MEASLES.

In these diseases, the diet should be about the same as in general fever. Plenty of water should be taken, or lemonade may be used, or weak tea. Not much strong food should be used until the patient is rapidly getting better, then rice plain or in puddings, farina, cup custards, sago, with cream or milk, baked apples, stewed prunes, then the meats that are allowed our patrons, and eggs.

INFLUENZA AND LA GRIPPE.

In these very common disorders, a fluid diet is the best at first or until the first violence of the attack is worn away. For the first two or three days milk is the best food. A patient may take as much as two quarts a day, without injury. After the fever subsides he may use beef, mutton or chicken broths, milk toast, custards, egg-nog, then stewed meats or a little broiled beef steak. Then, gradually, vegetables and the ordinary food.

DIPHTHERIA.

All foods must be given in a fluid form in cases of diphtheria. Of these, milk is the best, as usual. But it may be thickened with rice, cream or beaten eggs, using only the whites. Rice gruel is a splendid drink. Weak tea is allowed. After the fever is gone and the patient begins to recover, he may take broths, and arrowroot, rice, sago, etc., either plain or in puddings All toasts and gruels may be taken.

MALARIAL FEVERS.

In these fevers the diet should be about the same as that given under our general heading of diet in fevers. During the paroxysms of ague but little food of any kind should be taken. After these are over, especially when there is no fever present, if the patient has any appetite, he need not be quite as careful about his diet as in other cases of fever, but may take some solid food, if desired. But when the fever is on, the diet must be more carefully watched.

TUBERCULOSIS.

In this wasting disease, the food must be nutritious, and at the same time, it must be food that can be readily digested, and the stomach must be brought into condition to do its work. As we have already said, a small amount of food, which is digested, is of infinitely greater value to a sick person than a large amount of too strong food, which cannot be digested and simply remains in the stomach to ferment there, or is carried out of the body without doing the patient any good. For this reason, too often, highly-concentrated foods, such as cod-liver oil, blood, etc., etc., often do the consumptive patient no good, and he will gain flesh more rapidly upon a little rice, milk and other plain foods, if digested, than on all the beef extracts and cod liver oil in the world undigested. Our remedies help in the digestion of the food. They are foods in themselves, and our patrons very often gain flesh rapidly upon an exceedingly plain diet.

Still, patients of this class may vary their diet, if desired, much more than those suffering from wasting fevers or acute disorders. They may take barley, vermicelli or bouillon soups, vegetables soups, such as those prepared from peas, beans or celery. Milk either alone or in soups, may be used by some consumptives, but if there is much coughing or raising of phlegm, milk must be used sparingly. Whipped cream may be taken occasionally. Buttermilk may also be drank if acceptable to the patient. Fresh fish of any kind, preferably boiled. Eggs, soft-cooked, or in egg-nog or custard, poached or in plain omelet. All the meats that we have named in our bills of fare, chicken, turkeys, partridge, squab, or quail. Butter and olive oil may be used, the former on bread, the latter on lettuce.

For vegetables, we recommend baked potatoes, green peas, string beans, spinach, cooked celery, boiled onions, asparagus and cauliflower, but all vegetables must be used in moderation. All the cereals that we have recommended may be used; for fruits, baked or stewed apples, pears, prunes, grapes and blackberries, also stewed figs. Ripe olives may also be eaten by patients of this class.

Rice and bread puddings and blanc mange are good for desserts. Unfermented grape juice may be taken.

CHRONIC BRONCHITIS AND ASTHMA.

Patients suffering from asthma require great care in diet and should always avoid any tendency to overload the stomach. For any excess above the amount that can readily be digested, will cause fermentation and the accumulation of gases, which react upon the muscles of the diaphragm and abdomen and interfere with breathing, often causing distressing paroxysms. All food that is constipating or is likely to cause the formation of gas should be carefully avoided. All fats, sweets and starchy foods should be given up. No pork or veal should be used. No water should be taken with meals, or until three hours after a meal. A glass of hot water should be taken on rising in the morning and on retiring at night. All foods should be thoroughly masticated and patients suffering from these diseases should always be punctual in eating their meals at the same hours each day.

PNEUMONIA.

The general rules that we have given in severe cases of fever apply to cases of pneumonia and great care is necessary in the diet. All soups, liquors and stimulating foods must be strictly avoided. In this deadly disease the use of broths and liquors, under the delusion that they are sustaining the strength of the patient, is simply adding fuel to fire and is likely to burn out the life of the patient very quickly. The grease from broths goes to the lungs, burns there and fills them with a waste product which adds frightfully to the congestion and causes great danger. No starchy or sugary foods should be given. Plenty of cool drinks should be taken and milk should form the basis of the diet until the danger is past, and the fever is gone. Then other foods may be slowly added as given in our directions for cases of fever and recovery from fever.

ANAEMIA AND CHLOROSIS.

In these cases, the patient requires plenty of rest, and exercise in the open air, that is, moderate exercise. The strength should not be overtaxed. The diet should be liberal. Use plenty of milk, eggs and meat. Take hot water often.

FOO & WING HERB COMPANY

BRIGHT'S DISEASE.

Meats, eggs and all little made-up dishes are to be avoided in this disease. An exclusive milk diet is prescribed by American physicians and may be of benefit with our remedies. If the patient loses weight too rapidly under this, some farinaceous foods—that is, foods prepared from the different grains—may be added. Rice and bread are the best of these. In an exclusive milk diet, it is necessary to give from fourteen to eighteen or even twenty-two six-ounce glasses during each twenty-four hours. In some cases, milk does not agree and sours the stomach. If so, the quantity must be reduced. In ordinary cases, this diet must be continued for four to eight weeks. In some cases it may have to be followed out for six months or more. As the patient improves, boiled fish, chicken, game, butter cream and beef may be added, also olive oil. Tea and cocoa are permitted

We have never tied our patients down to so rigorous a diet, as our remedies act upon this disorder without that necessity. Still, we think that this diet is a good one for this disease and recommend it to all who have serious attacks of Bright's Disease.

GONORRHEA.

Persons afflicted with this acute disorder must avoid all starchy foods. In severe cases a diet of skimmed milk is the best at first. Then light farinaceous articles, such as rice, bread and butter, milk and some of the lighter cereals may be added. Alcoholic drinks must be strictly avoided. No acid fruits, fried foods, condiments can be used. Plenty of water should be drank, and soda, seltzer and apollinaris are all good.

TONSILITIS AND QUINSY.

In these diseases the food must be fluid and concentrated. Meat juice may be given, except when there is high fever, or beaten eggs; if necessary to make them appetizing a little brandy may be added to these. Milk is the best food in this disease as in so many others. A little plain vanilla ice cream may be given and is often soothing to the throat. It may also be used in cases of dyphtheria. As the patient improves, the diet should be more generous. Egg-nog and milk punch may be given and solid foods may be gradually added.

DYSPEPSIA.

There are so many forms of dyspepsia that it is almost impossible to give rules of diet that will apply in them all. Patients should follow our simple bills of fare. We give also the following general rules, which we have taken from a recent American work on diet:

1. Eat slowly and chew the food very thoroughly.
2. Drink fluids an hour before meals or two or three hours after meals rather than with meals.
3. Eat at regular hours.
4. If greatly fatigued lie down and rest before and after each meal.
5. Avoid, as far as possible, taking business worries or professional cares to the table.
6. Take systematic exercise in the open air. Walking, bicycle and horseback riding are the best forms.
7. If you are strong enough to bear a cold sponge bath, with vigorous friction by rough towels, on rising, this is advisable.
8. The bowels should be kept open by the use of laxative foods and fluids rather than by medicines.
9. Avoid too much variety at one meal. Take meats and vegetables at separate meals.

Weak tea in very hot water is often beneficial. Strong tea is astringent. Cocoa, but not chocolate, may be allowed to dyspeptics. Milk and vichy or milk and seltzer may be drank as a beverage, unless there is a tendency to flatulence. Avoid starchy foods, sweets, and milk and eggs if they disagree. Cream, fresh butter and olive oil are allowable.

DIARRHOEA.

Less food than the usual quantity taken, must be used in cases of diarrhoea. No irritating substances whatever should be taken into the stomach. No fruits, no vegetables. At the commencement of an acute attack, it is a good plan to go without food entirely for a day. Then give rice or arrowroot gruel or barley water. As the patient improves he may use mutton or chicken broth thickened, if desired, with boiled rice, tapioca, sago, arrowroot or cracker crumbs, or may take milk diluted with one-third rice water, if there is no vomiting. On returning to ordinary diet, first use such articles as milk toast, well-cooked macaroni, boiled rice, and baked or boiled potatoes. Rice gruel is very useful, both as a food and as a drink.

CHRONIC CONSTIPATION.

The vegetables allowed in our bills of fare should be freely used by persons suffering from chronic constipation, also coarse graham bread, rye bread, wheatena, wheat grits, Indian meal, oatmeal, Boston brown bread, olive oil, stewed figs, blueberries, apples, pears, prunes Fruit is most laxative when eaten between meals or half an hour before breakfast. The action of the fruit is assisted by drinking a tumberful or two of water. Two or three tumblerfuls of water either hot or cool, before retiring and on rising in the morning are also good. Also a tumberful about an hour after each meal. Foods to be avoided by persons with this trouble are eggs, milk, sweets, puddings, made from rice, sago, etc., all fried foods, gravies, sauces, strong coffee and tea.

HEMORRHOIDS.

Bulky foods should be avoided by persons suffering from hemorrhoids. Also milk. Fresh fruits should be eaten and aperient fluids taken. Regularity in meals and time of going to stool must be observed and abundant outdoor exercise taken.

ECZEMA.

In eczema the diet should be very simple. In bad cases a diet of milk, or bread and milk, for one, two or three weeks, is often of great benefit. From one and a half to two and a half quarts of milk may be taken each day. Meats of all kinds should be used very sparingly. Fish, boiled preferred, may be used sometimes. Tea, coffee, or cocoa not more than once a day, coffee not at all in severe cases. In some cases even oatmeal is too strong a food. Apples are not good in ecezma. The best food is whole wheat bread, fresh plainly-cooked vegetables, eggs, milk, and a little meat once a day. Do not take much fluid with meals.

OBESITY.

Hot water, taken half an hour before meals, on rising and on retiring, are beneficial and less fluid than otherwise is then required with the meals. Usually not more than five ounces of fluid should be taken with each meal, or fifteen ounces per day with meals, and this amount may be still further reduced by giving water between meals instead. Soups of all kinds are forbidden. Little milk should be used. The food should be as dry as possible, no watermelon or food like raw tomatoes should be eaten, no sugar, little fat, except butter, little farniaceous or starchy food. Gluten bread is better than wheat bread. Lean meat should form the basis of the diet, but should be varied with other foods.

DIET FOR LEANNESS.

Plenty of fat meats, butter, cream, milk, cocoa, chocolate, bread, potatoes, well-cooked cereals, especially oatmeal and cornmeal, farinaceous puddings—such as rice, sago and farina, with sugar and cream, sweets such as syrup and honey, sweet fruits. Avoid acids, sour fruits and fresh vegetables.

ACUTE RHEUMATISM.

While the fever lasts and other symptoms of acute disorder, such as pain and swelling of the joints, are present, the patient should be placed upon a fluid diet. Milk or bread and milk diet is best at these stages. If milk cannot be taken, then milk toast, rice, barley and oatmeal gruels and soups entirely free from fats may be used. Lemonade and slightly acid drinks may be taken, also weak tea. As the patient improves, the diet should be principally of farinaceous articles, but not starchy foods. Rice, arrowroot, oatmeal, cornmeal, wheat grits, milk toast, plain, unsweetened puddings, blanc mange are all good . No meat or fish for several days after the fever has subsided and the acute symptoms are gone. Later eggs, fish, a little lean meat, asparagus, spinach, stewed celery, baked apples and pears may be taken. No sweets, no alcohol under any circumstances, no malt liquors of any kind.

CHRONIC RHEUMATISM.

Not much meat; farinaceous foods and fresh green vegetables should be the basis of the diet, no sweets or alcoholic drinks. All foods should be thoroughly and plainly cooked and eaten in moderation.

DIABETES MELLITUS.

Foods permitted: Soups and broths made of lean meats and without vegetables, eggs, fresh fish, fresh meats, some chicken and turkey or game, olive oil, butter, cream, spinach, water cress, lettuce, asparagus, carrots, no sweet fruits, but some acid fruits such as sour apple, almonds, walnuts, Brazil nuts, hazel nuts, pecans.

Foods forbidden are sugar in any form, including honey, all starchy foods, such as rice, sago, tapioca, oatmeal, cornmeal, hominy, barley, macaroni, vermicelli, spaghetti, everything made of flour, all pastry, pies and puddings, such vegetables as beets, potatoes, parsley, peas, beans, turnips, cauliflower, rhubarb, sweet fruits, such as dates, figs, prunes, plums, bananas, apricots, berries of all kinds, chestnuts and peanuts. Use of water should be restricted, weak tea may be taken, either alone or with a little lemon, buttermilk may be drank, and plain soda or other mineral waters. Lithia waters are good.

NUTRITIOUS AND ATTRACTIVE DISHES FOR INVALIDS.

We give below recipes for preparing a number of dishes that will serve to tempt the appetite of invalids, and will prove of great value. Some of these are given after our own methods of cooking.

Others have been selected from various American books on cooking and diet. We give first the best methods of preparing food which, next to milk, is probably the best food in the world for most cases of sickness, namely, rice. This should always be the best quality obtainable and the best Chinese rice is the best in the world.

RICE GRUEL.

Take a quarter of a cup of rice and wash it until the water is clear. Boil it in six cupfuls of water for about one hour. A smaller quantity will cook in less time. Salt slightly. It is always to be taken warm. A cupful may be taken before each meal. It is excellent in case of cold and fever.

This preparation is very healthful and useful, especially for invalids and weakly persons. It is a splendid warm weather tonic, and cleanses and rinses out the stomach and removes the phlegm and residue, increases the juices and prepares the stomach for the meal.

The gruel quenches thirst when taken as herein directed; is also very soothing to all inflamed conditions of the internal organs, especially the stomach and bowels; also relieves indigestion and summer complaint. It is equally good for infants and invalids, and can be used to advantage by robust people. It should be used without dressing of any kind with infants who are in ill health, until a healthy condition of the system is reinstated. In hot weather the gruel should be made rather thin, but in cool weather it should be made as thick as mush. With people who are very feeble, a cupful of the gruel may be used two or three times daily in very warm weather, only a small quantity at a time.

There is no form of food that compares with this gruel as a tonic at all seasons of the year, for all people and in all conditions of ill health.

RICE WATER.

Thoroughly wash one ounce of rice in cold water. Then macerate for three hours in a quart of water kept at a tepid heat. Afterwards boil slowly for an hour. Then strain. This is a very useful drink in diarrhoea and dysentery and in all irritable states of the alimentary canal. It may be sweetened, or flavored with a little lemon peel, placed in the water while boiling, if desired.

ANOTHER RECIPE FOR RICE GRUEL.

Take two ounces of ground rice, one-fourth of an ounce of powdered cinnamon, four pints of water. Boil forty minutes and add one teaspoonful of orange marmalade.

RICE CREAM.

Two tablespoonfuls of rice, two cups of milk, one saltspoonful of salt, two tablespoonfuls of sugar, two eggs.

Cleanse the rice by washing it in several changes of cold water. Cook the rice with the milk in a double boiler until the grains will mash. Three hours will generally be required to do this. Should the milk evaporate, add more to make up for the amount lost. When the rice is thoroughly soft, press it through a colander or soup strainer into a saucepan. Return it to the fire, and while it is heating, beat the eggs, sugar and salt together until very light. When the rice boils, pour the eggs in slowly, stirring lightly with a spoon for three or four minutes or until the eggs and all coagulate, and the whole is like a thick, soft pudding. Then remove from the fire and pour it into a dish. By omitting the yolks of the eggs and using the whites only a delicate cream is obtained.

RICE AND APPLE.

Boil about two tablespoonfuls of rice in a pint and a half of new milk, stirring it from time to time until the rice is quite tender. Have ready some apples, peeled, cored and stewed to a pulp, and sweetened, with a very little loaf sugar. Put the rice around the plate, and the apples in the middle and serve.

DIRECTIONS FOR COOKING PLAIN RICE.

Wash one cup of rice till the water runs clear; then add two cups of cold water and boil in a stewpan till the rice appears to be boiled about dry—till the rice shows holes in the top or settles in places—which will appear in about fifteen minutes after the boiling commences. Then the stewpan should be placed on the stove where the heat is low, and allowed to steam about twenty minutes, or until the rice is thoroughly, cooked and very soft, so that the kernels will mash easily. A cloth should be placed over the stewpan and the cover over that when the stewpan is placed to steam, for the purpose of retaining the steam in the stewpan. Do not stir the rice but once, and then within a few minutes after it commences to boil. When well cooked the rice should be very light and lay up loose, and each kernel appear to be ready to roll away from the others. It should be eaten in the state that it comes from the stewpan.

Rice cooked in the above manner should constitute one-half of the meals regularly, at least twice each day. By using the rice as a base food, one is not at all likely to over eat, or eat more than the powers of digestion can work up perfectly.

We never have known of an instance where a person who persisted in the use of rice cooked in the way prescribed above, did not become attached to the article and feel that they could not make a meal without it, and really prefer it to bread or potatoes.

A heavy iron porcelained-lined stewpan is best, and agate ware is second best to cook rice in.

TO COOK RICE QUICKLY.

Rice may be cooked very thoroughly and well in half an hour if attention is paid to the details of the process, so as to secure all the benefit of the steam that is generated while the rice is cooking. Take one cup of rice and two cups of water. The cups may be larger or smaller as desired. First wash the rice very thoroughly, in four changes of water. Pour the two cups of water over it, in an agate stewpan or pail, covered tightly. Put it over a fire, either a stove or an alcohol or gasoline fire. In ten minutes it will commence to boil. Let it boil hard for about ten minutes without stirring or opening the dish. At first when there is a greater amount of steam, it will spurt out of the edges of the cover. As the steam grows less it will come slower and will rise nearly straight into the air. This is an indication that the rice has boiled long enough, but, in any event, from eight to twelve minutes is the proper time.

Now take the dish from the fire, and let it stand a few minutes, say about five, where it will partially cool. The steam in the top of the pail and the moisture will condense and settle to the bottom. Do not remove the lid. After a few minutes place the rice carefully over the fire, turning the dish so that the fire will not be long in one place, and let this condensed moisture be boiled away. Only two or three minutes will be required for this. Then remove from the fire, still with the cover on, and let the dish stand five or ten minutes longer, so that the steam and hot air still in the dish above the rice will cook it on top. Then remove the cover and you will find the rice thoroughly cooked, dry and the kernels unbroken. Sprinkle with salt and eat plain, or with a little butter.

TO COOK EGGS.

Take the whites of two eggs, well beaten, and two tablespoonfuls of cold boiled water, and salt to suit taste; place the bowl in a stewpan of boiling water, then cover the stewpan in a manner to confine the steam. Cook about twenty minutes, or until thoroughly done.

For the first few days, use every other day, then once daily. All may be eaten at one time, using other foods to complete the meal.

By using cold boiled water, it will dissolve the eggs and there will be no lumps. If you should prefer them thinner, add more water.

ANOTHER GOOD WAY TO COOK EGGS.

The following is an excellent way to cook eggs, when patients are sufficiently strong to digest eggs boiled in the ordinary way:

Have ready a small pail, or covered dish, filled with boiling water. A quart pail will be large enough for three eggs, a gallon for eight or ten. Place the eggs in the boiling water and cover tight. Set them aside, away from the fire for fifteen minutes. In this way the eggs are all cooked evenly and after a little experimenting, any one can learn how long to cook them in order to have them done just right.

EGG TIMBALES.

A Very Dainty and Attractive Dish, Either for Invalids or Well People.

To prepare these properly, one should have little tin or agate ware cups so that they may be made as small as desired. But ordinary tea or coffee cups will answer. Old cups with the handles broken are good enough. Grease the cups with melted butter. Beat four eggs, whites and yolks together and add a pinch of salt and a cup of milk. Fill the little cups, place them in a pan and fill the pan with boiling water to half way up the sides of the cups. Bake in the oven from ten to fifteen minutes, trying them with a silver knife as you would a custard. When they cease to stick to the knife they are done. Prepare a cream sauce by taking one tablespoonful of butter melted in a dish. Stir in a tablespoonful of flour and let it dissolve. Then add one and a fourth cups of milk, a teaspoonful of salt, and stir it over the fire, boiling until it thickens. Turn out the timbales of egg on a hot dish and cover with the hot cream sauce. Serve hot. These are very appetizing and very nutritious; should not be made too large for an invalid.

A NUTRITIOUS WAY OF PREPARING MUSHES.

Germea, cream of wheat and similar finely-ground cereals may be cooked and served in a very digestible and nutritious mush in the following way: Take one pint of water and one pint of milk. To this and three-fourths of a cup of the wheat or germea and one teaspoonful of salt Bring these to the boiling point, then stir in the wheat slowly till the mush thickens. Cook for an hour, if possible in a double boiler.

BARLEY WATER.

Take two ounces of pearl barley and wash well in cold water, putting through two or three washings. Afterwards boil in a pint and a half of water or twenty minutes in a covered vessel. Strain. The resulting liquid may be sweetened and flavored with lemon peel, or lemon peel may be added while the boiling is going on, to give it a little flavor. This makes a soothing and mildly nutritive drink something like rice gruel.

ANOTHER RECIPE FOR BARLEY WATER.

Wash two ounces of pearl barley in cold water. Then boil it for five minutes in some fresh water and throw both waters away. Then pour on two quarts of boiling water and boil it down to one quart.

Stir and skim occasionally. Flavor with finely cut lemon peel, add sugar to taste, but do not strain unless the patient prefers it strained.

MULLED WINE.

Although we do not very often permit our patients wine or any other drink containing alcohol, yet it is possible that there might be some circumstances under which it would be allowable. We, therefore, give the following receipt for mulled wine:

Boil down spices, cloves, nutmeg, cinnamon or mace, in a little water, just to flavor the wine. Then add a wineglassful or two of sherry or any other wine, and bring it to a boil. Serve with little pieces of toast. Sweeten, if desired. If claret is used it will require some sugar. The vessel in which this is boiled should be absolutely clean.

LEMONADE.

Pare the rind from a lemon thinly and cut the lemon into slices. Put the peel and the sliced lemon into a pitcher with one ounce of white sugar. Pour over them one pint of boiling water. Cover the pitcher closely and let stand until cool enough to drink. Strain or pour off the liquid. May be taken hot or cool.

BEEF JUICE.

Broil quickly some pieces of round or sirloin of beef of a size to fit into the cavity of a lemon squeezer previously heated by being dipped into hot water. The juice, as it runs away from the squeezer should be received into a wine glass and, after being seasoned to taste with salt and cayenne pepper, should be taken while hot.

BEEF ESSENCE.

Cut a lean piece of beef into small pieces and place them in a wide-mouthed bottle, securely corked, and allow it to stand for several hours in a vessel of boiling water. This may sometimes be used when it is important that the patient should have considerable nourishment, and milk disagrees with the stomach.

BEEF TEA.

Chop fine a pound of lean beef, free from fat, tissues, gristle, etc., cover with a pint of cold water, and let stand for two hours. Then let it simmer on the stove for three hours at a temperature never over 160 deg. Make up the water lost through evaporation by adding cold water so that when done, one pint of beef tea will represent a pound of beef. Strain and carefully express all the fluid from the beef.

CHICKEN BROTH.

Skin and chop up into small pieces a small chicken or half of a larger one, and boil it, bones and all, with a blade of mace, a sprig of parsley and a crust of bread in a quart of water for an hour, skimming it from time to time to take off all the fat and scum. Then strain through a colander.

CHICKEN, VEAL OR MUTTON BROTH.

Chicken, veal or mutton broth may be made like beef tea by substituting chicken, veal or mutton for beef, boiling in a sauce pan for two hours and straining. For chicken broth, the bones should be crushed and added. For veal broth the fleshy part of the knuckle should be used. Either of these broths may be thickened and its nutritive value increased by adding pearl barley, rice, vermicelli or macaroni.

BEEF TEA WITH OATMEAL.

This makes a very nutritious food. Take two tablespoonfuls of oatmeal and two of cold water and mix them thoroughly. Then add a pint of good beef tea which has just been brought to the boiling point. Boil together for five minutes stirring it well all the time, and strain through a sieve.

MILK AND CINNAMON DRINK.

Boil with one pint of new milk, sufficient cinnamon to flavor it pleasantly and sweeten with white sugar. This may be taken cold with a teaspoonful of brandy and is very good for diarrhoea. Children may take it warm without the brandy.

MILK PUNCH

Is made by adding brandy, or whiskey, or rum to milk in the proportion of about one part of liquor to four or six parts of milk. Flavor with sugar and nutmeg and shake well. Will not often be required by our patients.

HOME-MADE LIME WATER.

Pour two quarts of hot water over fresh, unslacked lime (a piece the size of a walnut). Stir until it is slacked, then let it stand until it becomes clear and bottle it. This is often added to milk to neutralize the acidity of the stomach.

EGG-NOG.

Is made by adding the beaten yolks of eggs and a little spirits to a tumberful of milk, stirring well, and adding sugar and the whites of the eggs separately beaten. One egg is usually sufficient, the digestibility of this food is greatly increased by adding half an ounce of lime water which does not affect the taste at all.

ANOTHER WAY.

Scald down new milk by putting it contained in a jug into a sauce pan of boiling water, but it must not be allowed to boil. When the milk is cold, beat up an egg in a tumbler with a fork, together with a little sugar. Beat it to a froth. Add a dessert-spoonful of brandy and fill up the tumbler with some of the scalded milk. This is a nutritive drink in some acute diseases where there is no fever.

ARROWROOT BLANC MANGE.

This makes a good light dessert for invalids. Take two table-spoonsful of arrowroot, three fourths of a pint of milk, lemon and sugar to taste. Mix the arrowroot with a little milk into a smooth batter. Pour the rest of the milk over this; put on the fire and let it boil, sweeten and flavor it, stirring all the time until it thickens sufficiently. Put into a mould until it is quite cold.

ARROWROOT.

Mix thoroughly two teaspoonfuls of arrowroot in three tablespoonfuls of cold water and then pour on these, half a pint of boiling water, stirring well meanwhile. If the water is quite boiling, the arrowroot thickens and it is poured off and nothing more is necessary. If only warm water is used, the arrowroot must afterwards be boiled until it thickens. Sweeten with loaf sugar, and flavor with lemon peel or nutmeg or with sherry wine, or with port wine or brandy if desired. Boiling milk may be used instead of the water, but when this is done, no wine or spirits must be used or it will curdle.

OATMEAL GRUEL.

Take one tablespoonful of oatmeal, one saltspoonful of salt, one scant teaspoonful of sugar, one cupful of boiling water, one cupful of milk. Mix the oatmeal, salt and sugar together and pour on the boiling water. Cook for thirty minutes. Then strain through a fine wire strainer to remove the hulls of the oatmeal. Place again on the stove, add the milk and let it come just to the boiling point. Serve hot

SCOTCH BEEF BROTH.

To a pint of beef broth which has been carefully strained and seasoned, and from which all fat has been removed, add a teaspoonful of oatmeal and boil gently for two hours. Strain and serve hot. In this preparation the oatmeal should be soft and jelly-like, and if too much water evaporates during the boiling, more should be added.

SOME POINTS ON COOKING.

The main thing to remember in regard to all forms of cooking for invalids, is that everything must be very thoroughly cooked for the purpose of rendering it easily digestible. This applies equally to bread, cereals, meats and vegetables. In our opinion, the best way to cook foods for invalids is by steaming them, boiling is next best. We rarely permit our patrons to eat anything that is broiled or roasted, although for the sake of variety, we may occasionally permit a little roast beef, or baked potatoes or broiled meats, such as bacon, chicken or beefsteak. The reason for this is that foods cooked in hot air are too dry. They do not supply the juices of the system but, on the other hand, exhaust those juices upon which digestion and health depend. This is a point, we think, not fully understood by American writers on diet.

Double boilers are the best dishes for cooking, so that the food may be inclosed in one dish and surrounded by hot water contained in the other dish. A gas fire is very fine, because the heat may be regulated so as to cook the food thoroughly and evenly. The best way to prepare cream or milk, is to steam it in the following way. Place the milk or cream in a boiler or dish and set that boiler or dish into another containing boiling water, and allow the water to boil until the milk or cream has been thoroughly cooked. For milk or cream, the cover on the inside dish should be perforated to permit the steam to escape.

All meats, mushes, cereals and vegetables may be cooked in the same way, but inside dish should have a tight cover to confine the steam and the cooking should be slow but thorough. Meats and vegetables should be steamed with just enough water to cover them. adding more, from time to time, if necessary and, in the case of meats, the resulting juices form a very nutritious and palatable gravy, containing all the nutriment. A piece of tender beefsteak cut into small pieces, covered with water, and steamed in this way until well cooked, say for an hour, makes a most palatable dish. Ducks and chickens may be cooked in the same way and served with boiled rice and green peas, are splendid. Serve the gravy with the rice. There is no danger of cooking too thoroughly.

All vegetables must be thoroughly cooked and in enough water to make them soft without being sloppy. Such articles of food as rice, oatmeal, wheat flakes and potatoes need very thorough cooking by steaming or boiling to break up the starch granules and render them fit for taking into the human stomach. If these granules are not well cooked, they are hard and indigestible, but, if well cooked, as in a nicely-baked or boiled potato, or in well-cooked rice, they burst apart and are readily converted into sugar during the digestive processes and this, in turn, is digested and goes to nourish and strengthen the individual. This breaking apart of the starch granules is what gives the attractive, "mealy" appearance to a well-cooked potato, as distinguished from the hard, clammy, soggy appearance of a half-cooked potato or one that has been allowed to stand in water after the cooking was finished.

The following remarks upon the cooking of meats are taken from one of the bulletins issued by the United States Department of Agriculture for the benefit of the people at large and are quoted here because they agree with our ideas upon this subject. The following ideas are given upon the subject of boiling meats:

"If meat is placed in cold water, part of the organic salts, the soluble albumen and the extractives or flavoring matters will be dissolved out. At the same time small portions of lactic acid are formed; which act upon the meat and change some of the insoluble matters into materials which may also be dissolved out. The extent of this action and the quantity of materials which actually go into the solution depend upon three things; the amount of surface exposed to the water, the temperature of the water, and the length of the time of the exposure. The smaller the pieces, the longer the time, or the hotter the water, the richer will be the broth and the poorer the meat. If the water is heated gradually more and more of the soluble materials are dissolved.

"If, on the other hand, a piece of meat is plunged into boiling water, the albumen on the entire surface of the meat is quickly coagulated and the enveloping crust thus formed resists the dissolving action of water and prevents the escape of the juices and flavoring matters. Thus cooked, the meat retains most of its flavoring matters, and has the desired meaty taste. The resulting broth is correspondingly poor.

"The foregoing statements will be of much help in the rational cooking of meats in water. The treatment depends largely upon what it is desired to do. It is impossible to make a rich broth and have a juicy, highly-flavored piece of boiled meat at the same time. If the meat alone is to be used the cooking in water should be as follows: Plunge the cut at once into a generous supply of boiling water and keep the water at the boiling point, or as near boiling as possible, for ten minutes, in order to coagulate the albumen and seal the pores of the meat; the coating thus formed will prevent the solvent action of the water and the escape of the soluble albumen and juices from the inner portions of the meat. But if the action of the boiling water should be continued, the whole interior of the meat would, in time, be brought near the temperature of boiling water, and all the albumen would be coagulated and rendered hard. Instead of keeping the water at the boiling point, (212 deg.,) therefore the temperature should be allowed to fall to about 180 deg., when the meat could be thoroughly cooked without becoming hard. A longer time will be required for cooking meat in this way, but the albumen will not be firmly coagulated, and the flesh will be tender and juicy instead of tough and dry, as will be the case when the water is kept boiling, or nearly boiling, during the entire time of cooking."

STEWING.

"If both the broth and the meat are to be used, the process of cooking should be quite different from that outlined for boiling meat. Stewing is in this country, a much undervalued method of cooking. This is probably partly due to the fact that stewing is generally very improperly done.

"In stewing, the meat should be cut into small pieces, so as to present relatively as large a surface as possible, and, instead of being quickly plunged into hot water, should be put into cold water in order that much of the juices and flavoring materials may be dissolved. The temperature should then be slowly raised until it reaches about 180 deg. F., where it should be kept for some hours. Treated in this way, the broth will be rich and the meat still tender and juicy.

"If the water is made much hotter than 180 deg. F., the meat will be dry and fibrous. It is true that if a high temperature is maintained long enough the connective tissues will be changed to gelatine and partly dissolved away, and the meat will apparently be so tender that if touched with a fork it will fall to pieces. It will be discovered, however, that no matter how easily the fibers come apart, they offer considerable resistance to mastication. The albumen and fibrin have become thoroughly coagulated, and while the fibers have separated from each other the prolonged boiling has only made them drier and firmer."

STEAMING, THE BEST WAY TO COOK MEATS.

It will be seen from the above quotations, that, according to the highest American authority, stewing, or slowly-cooking meats, commencing with cold water and gradually heating it to a point where it will simmer but not boil, is the best way, when both the meat and the broth is to be used as food. But, in our opinion, the method of steaming, in a double boiler, covering the meat with only a little cold water, which is heated into steam, is still better. Our patients should use whichever of these ways is most convenient, as a general rule, in cooking meats, and should employ other ways only occasionally, and as a matter of variety.

BROTHS, SOUPS AND MEAT EXTRACTS.

The same authority that we have already quoted has the following to say upon the subject of broths, soups and meat extracts, and the reader will note that these remarks fully sustain the position that we have always held in regard to the use of soups and broths in cases of fever and other acute diseases, namely, that the use of such foods is a source of the greatest danger, and is likely to imperil the patient's life. The article says:

"The quantities of ingredients in a meat broth may be illustrated by a German experiment. One pound of beef and seven ounces of veal bones gave about a pint of strong broth or soup, which contained, by weight, water 95.2 per cent.; protien, 1.2 per cent.; fat 1.5 per cent.; extractives, 1.8 per cent.; mineral matters .3 per cent.

"Very palatable broths can be made by using more water and adding savory herbs. Broths thus made, have, of course, a greater amount of water, frequently as much as 98 per cent. or even more, and the nutrients are correspondingly reduced in amount. It would appear from the analysis given above, that the amount of solids in broths is generally small. Consequently their strong taste and stimulating effect upon the nervous system must be ascribed to the meat bases (flavoring matters) and to the salts of potash which they contain. Besides meat bases soups contain more or less gelatine, varying directly with the quantity of bones used in the preparation.

"The true meat extract, if pure, contains little else besides the flavoring matters of the meat from which it is prepared, together with such mineral salts as may be dissolved out. It should contain no gelatine or fat, and cannot, from the way in which it is made, contain any albumen. It is, therefore, not a food at all but a stimulant, and should be classed with tea, coffee, and other allied substances. It should never be administered to the sick except as directed by competent medical advice. Its strong, meaty taste is deceptive, and the person depending upon it alone for food would certainly die of starvation. Broth and beef tea as prepared ordinarily in the household contain more or less protein, gelatine and fat, and, therefore, are foods as well as stimulants. The proportion of water in such compounds is always very large."

The reader will see at once that the above bears out the contention which we have maintained for many years, namely, that broths, meat extracts and rich soups of all kinds are not true foods but stimulants and therefore harmful in fevers. The object of the American physician in the treatment of fevers is different from ours. He wishes to maintain the strength of the patient until the disease has run its course. We desire to develop the juices of the system and to drown out the fever at the start, not permitting it to run its course. Therefore, although the use of stimulants may be perfectly proper from the point of view of the American doctor, it is exactly contrary to our teachings. Our patrons need not fear starvation during the few hours required for our remedies to do their work and to lessen the fever. Be content with a little of the plainest food, rice, milk and similar articles for a few days. The fever will then be less and stronger nourishment may be employed safely. We have given some receipts for broths and soups, but we wish to impress, once more, upon our patrons the fact that these are to be used with the greatest caution in all critical cases.

THE PROPER WAY TO COOK FISH.

The best fish for the use of invalids are those that are white-meated, cod, halibut, barracouda, etc. Salmon and dark-meated fish are too strong. The best way to cook these is by boiling. But the water should not be boiling when the fish are put into it. Let it be on the point of boiling and kept at this temperature for a few minutes, then permit it to fall to a temperature of about 180 deg. Cooking from twenty to thirty minutes in water at this temperature will usually be sufficient. Serve with a plain cream sauce.

A WORD IN CONCLUSION.

In conclusion of these directions on cooking we can only repeat what we have already said. Be very careful of your diet, eat the plainest foods and never overeat. Run the risk of eating too little rather than too much and give our herbal remedies a chance to restore the stomach to its normal activities before you burden it with much food. This is altogether the safest course. The withdrawal of tea, coffee and stimulating foods from your diet may give you a sensation of weakness and languor for a short time. But this will soon pass away and you will then be surprised to see how much strength you will derive from plain food thoroughly digested. In this fact lies half the secret of a cure. And we cannot repeat this caution too often or too emphatically.

DIET IN HEALTH.

The Uses of Food in the Human Body.

We do not desire to leave our patrons, after recovery, entirely without advice upon the subject of what they shall eat, one of the most important questions that any person has to consider. As a general rule, patrons of our system who have been restricted in their use of foods for several months naturally wish, after recovery, to allow themselves some greater freedom in their choice of foods. To this we do not strongly object, provided that caution and common sense are exercised. But we propose to show, under this heading, that the diet which we have laid down for invalids is also, in a sense, the best for well persons, that is to say the articles selected for invalids should also form the basis of the diet for well people, and any additions or variations should be made with caution. Many people find our diet so wholesome and beneficial that they have little desire to depart from it, to any great extent, after they are beyond the further need of taking the medicines.

As we are discussing American foods, and not Chinese foods, we have tried to adapt our ideas to American ways of living, as far as possible. And we have taken the following remarks upon the use of foods from a very valuable book on diet entitled "Practical Dietetics" by Gilman Thompson, M.D., recently published by D. Appleton & Co., of New York. We do not agree with many of Mr. Thompson's ideas, yet there are many suggestions in his book which are of great value. On the subject of the use of foods by the human body, he says:

"The two ultimate uses of all food are to supply the body with materials for growth or renewal and with energy for the capacity for doing work. The energy received in a latent form, stored in the various chemical combinations of foods, is liberated as kinetic or active energy in two chief forms, first as heat, second as motion. Force is a manifestation of energy. The force developed by a healthy adult at ordinary labor, averages 3400 foot tons per day, a foot ton being the amount of force required to raise a weight of one ton through the height of one foot. Of this, somewhat less than one-fifth is expended in motion and somewhat more than four-fifths, or 2840 foot tons, in heat, which maintains the body temperature at its normal average.

"A man weighing 150 pounds, or over one-thirteenth of a ton, obviously expends considerable energy in merely moving his own body about from place to place, aside from carrying any additional burden. The original force developed in the various functions of animal life, which results in heat production and motion, is chiefly obtained from the radiant heat of the sun stored in plants in the latent form of certain chemical combinations, chiefly starches and sugars, which, by being consumed as food by animals, furnish energy."

This subject is further illustrated by the following comparison of the human body with a steam engine, which we have taken from an old scrap book. It gives a very clear description, in language which everybody can understand, of the way in which the food that is eaten by man is converted into the various uses necessary to sustain life. It is entitled,

THE BODY AND ITS COMPOSITION.

"The lamp of life" is a very old metaphor for the mysterious principle vitalizing nerve and muscle, but no other comparison could be so apt. The full-grown adult takes in each day, through lungs and mouth, about eight and a half pounds of dry food, water, and the air necessary for breathing purposes. Through the pores of the skin, the lungs, kidneys, and lower intestines, there is a corresponding waste, and both supply and waste amount in a year to one and a half tons, or three thousand pounds.

The steadiness and clear shining of the flame of a lamp depend upon quality as well as amount of the oil supplied, and, too, the texture of the wick; and so all human life and work are equally made or marred by the food which sustains life, as well as the nature of the constitution receiving that food.

Before the nature and quality of food can be considered, we must know the constitutents of the body to be fed, and something of the process through which digestion and nutrition are accomplished.

I shall take for granted that you have a fairly plain idea of the stomach and its dependences. Physiologies can always be had, and for minute details they must be referred to. Bear in mind one or two main points; that all food passes from the mouth to the stomach, an irregularly-shaped pouch or bag with an opening into the duodenum, and from thence into the larger intestine. Fom the mouth to the end of this intestine, the whole may be called the alimentary canal, is a tube of varying size and some thirty-six feet in length. The mouth must be considered part of it, as it is in the mouth that digestion actually begins, all starchy foods depending upon the action of the saliva for genuine digestion, saliva having some strange power by which starch is converted into sugar. Swallowed whole or placed directly in the stomach, such food passes through the body unchanged. Each division of the alimentary canal has its own distinct digestive juice, and I give them in the order in which they occur.

First. The saliva, secreted from the glands of the mouth; alkaline, glairy, adhesive.

Second. The gastric juice, secreted in the inner or third lining of the stomach, an acid, and powerful enough to dissolve all the fibre and albumen of flesh food.

Third. The pancreatic juice, secreted by the pancreas, which you know in animals as sweetbreads. The juice has a peculiar influence upon fats, which remain unchanged by saliva and gastric juice, and not until dissolved by pancreatic juice, and made into what chemists call an emulsion, can they be absorbed into the system.

Fourth. The bile, which no physiologist as yet thoroughly understands. We know its action, but hardly why it acts. It is a necessity, however, for if by disease the supply be cut off, an animal emaciates and soon dies.

Fifth. The intestinal juice, which has some properties like saliva, and is the last product of the digestive forces.

A meal, then, in its passage downward is first diluted and increased in bulk by a watery fluid which prepares all the starchy portion for absorption. Then comes a still more profuse fluid, dissolving all the meaty part. Then the fat is attended by the stream of pancreatic juice, and at the same time the bile pours upon it, doing its own work in its own mysterious way; and last of all, lest any process should have been imperfect, the long canal sends out a juice having some of the properties of all.

Thus each day's requirements call for:

	Grammes.
Of saliva	3 3-4
Of gastric juice	12
Of bile	3 3-4
Of pancreatic juice	1 1-2
Of intestinal juice	1-2
	21 1-2

Do not fancy this is all wasted or lost. Very far from it; for the whole process seems to be a second circulation, as it were; and while the blood is moving in its wonderful passage through veins and arteries, another circulation as wonderful, an endless current going its unceasing round so long as life lasts, is also taking place. But without food the first would become impossible; and the quality of food, and its proper digestion, mean good or bad blood as the case may be. We must follow our mouthful of food, and see how this action takes place.

When the different juices have all done their work the chyme, which is food as it passes from the stomach into the duodenum or passage to the lower stomach or bowels, becomes a milky substance called chyle, which moves slowly, pushed by numberless muscles along the bowel, which squeeze much of it into little glands at the back of the bowels. These are called the mesentric glands; and, as each one receives its portion of chyle, a wonderful thing happens. About half of it is changed into small, round bodies called corpuscles, and they float with the rest of the milky fluid through delicate pipes which take it to a sort of bag just in front of the spine. To this bag is fastened another pipe or tube—the thoracic duct—which follows the line of the spine; and up this tube the small bodies travel till they come to the neck and a spot where two veins meet. A door in one opens and the transformation is complete. The small bodies are raw food no more, but blood, traveling fast to where it may be purified, and begin its endless round in the best condition. For, as you know, venous blood is still impure and dirty blood. Before it can be really alive it must pass through the veins to the right side of the heart, flow through into the upper chamber, then through another door or valve into the lower, where it is pumped out into the lungs. If these lungs are, as they should be, full of pure air, each corpuscle is so charged with oxygen that the last speck of impurity is burned up, and it goes dancing and bounding on its way. That is what health means; perfect food made into perfect blood, and giving that sense of strength and exhilaration that we none of us know half as much about as we should. We get it sometimes on mountain-tops in clear autumn days when the air is like wine, but nature meant it to be our daily portion, and this very despised knowledge of cookery is to bring it about. If a lung is imperfect, supplied only with foul air as among the very poor, or diseased as in consumption, food does not nourish, and you now know why. We have found that the purest air and the purest water contain the largest proportion of oxygen; and it is this that vitalizes the food and, through food the blood.

To nourish this body then demands many elements; and to study these has been the joint work of chemists and physiologists, till at last every constituent of the body is known and classified. Many as these constituents are, they are all resolved into the simple elements, oxygen, hydrogen, nitrogen and carbon, while a little sulphur, a little phosphorus, lime, chlorine, sodium, etc., are added.

Flesh and blood are composed of water, fat, fibrine, albumen, gelatine, and the compounds of lime, phosphorus, soda, potash, magnesia, iron, etc.

Bone contains cartilage, gelatine, fat, and the salts of lime, magnesia, soda, etc., in combination with phosphoric and other acids.

Cartilage consists of chondrine, a substance somewhat like gelatine, and contains all the salts of sulphur, lime, soda, potash, phosphorus, magnesia and iron.

Bile is made up of water, fat, resin, sugar, cholesterine, some fatty acids, and the salts of potash, iron and soda.

The Brain is made up of water, albumen, fat, phosphoric acid, osmazone and salts.

The Liver unites water, fat and albumen with phosphoric and other acids, and lime, iron, soda and potash.

The Lungs are formed of two substances: one like gelatine, another of the nature of caseine and albumen, fibrine, cholesterine, iron, water, soda, and various fatty and organic acids.

How these varied elements are held together, even science with all its deep searchings has never told. No man, by whatever combination of elements, has ever made a living plant, much less a living animal. No better comparison has ever been given than that of Youmans, who makes a table of the analogies between the human body and the steam engine, which I give as it stands:

ANALOGIES OF THE STEAM ENGINE AND THE LIVING BODY.

The steam engine in action takes:

1. Fuel: Coal and wood, both combustible.
2. Water for evaporation
3. Air for combustion.

And Produces:

4. A steady boiling heat of 212 degs. by quick combustion.
5. Smoke loaded with carbonic acid and watery vapor.
6. Combustible ashes.
7. Motive force of simple alternate push and pull in the piston, which, acting through wheels, bands and levers, does work of endless variety.
8. A deficiency of fuel, water or air, disturbs, then stops the motion.

The animal body in life takes:

1. Food: Vegetables and flesh, both combustible.
2. Water for circulation.
3. Air for respiration.

And Produces:

4. A steady animal heat by slow combustion of 98 deg.
5. Expired breath loaded with carbonic acid and watery vapor.
6. Combustible animal refuse.
7. Motive force of simple alternate contraction and relaxation in the muscles which, acting through joints, tendons and levers, does work of endless variety.
8. A deficiency of food, drink or air first disturbs, then stops the motion and the life.

Carrying out this analogy you will at once see why a person working hard with either body or mind requires more food than the one who does but little. The food taken into the human body can never be a simple element. We do not feed on plain, undiluted oxygen or nitrogen; and, while the composition of the human body includes really sixteen elements in all, oxygen is the only one used in its natural state. I give first the elements as they exist in a body weighing about one hundred and fifty pounds, this being the average weight of a full-grown man; and add a table, compiled from different sources, of the composition of the body as made up from these elements. Dry as such details may seem, they are the only key to a full understanding of the body, and the laws of the body, so far as the food supply is concerned; though you will quickly find that the day's food means the day's thought and work, well or ill, and that in your hands is put a power mightier than you know—the power to build up body, and through body the soul, into a strong and healthful manhood and womanhood.

COMPOSITION OF THE BODY.

		Lbs.	Ozs.	Grs.
1.	Water, which is found in every part of the body and amounts to	109	0	0
2.	Fibrine and like substances, found in the blood and forming the chief solid materials of the flesh	15	10	0
3.	Phosphate of lime, chiefly in bones and teeth, but in all liquids and tissues	8	12	0
4.	Fat, a mixture of three chemical compounds, and distributed all through the body	4	8	0
5.	Osseine, the organic framework of bones; boiled gives gelatine; weight	4	7	350
6.	Keratine, a nitrogenous substance, forming the greater part of hair, nails and skin, weighs	4	2	0
7.	Cartilagine resembles the osseine of bone, and is a nitrogenous substance, the chief constituent of cartilage, weighing	1	8	0
8.	Haemoglobine gives the red color to blood, and is a nitrogenous substance, containing iron, and weighing	1	8	0
9.	Albumen is a soluble nitrogenous substance, found in the blood; chyle, lymph and muscle, and weighs	1	1	0
10.	Carbonate of lime is found in the bones chiefly, and weighs	1	1	0
11.	Hephalin is found in nerves and brain, with cerebrine and other compounds	0	13	0
12.	Fluoride of calcium is found in teeth and bones, and weighs	0	7	175
13.	Phosphate of magnesia is also in teeth and bones, and weighs	0	7	0
14.	Chloride of sodium, or common salt, is found in all parts of the body	0	7	0
15.	Cholesterine, glycogen and inosite are compounds containing hydrogen, oxygen and carbon, found in muscle, liver and brain, and weighing	0	3	0

16. Sulphate phosphate and salts of sodium, found in all tissues and liquids 0 2 107
17. Sulphate, phosphate and chloride of potassium are also in all tissues and liquids.................... 0 0 300
18. Silica, found in hair, skin and bones................ 0 0 30

                              154 0 0

SUBSTANCES THAT CAN BE USED AS FOOD.

Having thus given our readers some idea of the way that food is employed in the human body to sustain life and to permit the body to perform its functions, we now come to the question, "What are food elements?" In other words, "what are the substances that the body takes up and appropriates to undergo the different chemical changes necessary to make blood, bone, flesh, brain and sinew?" Upon this point we give the following chart which shows at a glance the primary materials into which all food is reduced. This is one of the charts published by the United States Government and prepared by its eminent expert, Professor Wilbur Olin Atwater. Here it is:

Food Materials as Purchased.	Edible Portions, Flesh of Meat, Yolk and White of Eggs, Wheat, Flour, Etc.	Water, Nutrients,	Protein, Fats, Carbohydrates, Mineral Matter.
	Refuse, Bones, Entrails, Shells, Etc.		

Protein forms tissues, i. e., muscle, tendon and fat.
 White of eggs, i. e., albumen; curd of milk, i. e., **casein; lean** meat, gluten of wheat, etc.
Fats form fatty tissues.
 Fat of meat, butter, olive oil, oils of corn and wheat, etc.
Carbohydrates:
 Sugar, starch, etc., are transformed into fats.

Mineral Matters aid in forming bones, assist in digestion, etc.

Phosphate of lime, potash, soda, etc.

All of the above, the protein, the fats, the carbohydrates and the mineral matters serve as fuel and yield energy in the form of heat and muscular strength.

DEFINITION OF PROTEIN.

Perhaps the word protein is sufficiently explained above by showing the shapes in which it appears, in its purest form, as food. Yet it occurs so frequently in all works on diet that perhaps the chemical definition will not be out of place. It is as follows: Protein is a compound obtained from proteids, originally regarded as a proteid deprived of its sulphur, but now as an artificial product resembling alkali albumen.

It appears that, in order to know what protein is, we must also know what a proteid is, and the definition of this latter is as follows:

Proteid, any one of a class of highly complex and usually amorphous compounds containing carbon, hydrogen, oxygen, nitrogen and sulphur, found as viscous solids or in solution in nearly all the solids and liquids of animal and vegetable organisms.

Proteids are the most important animal and vegetable compounds, and none of the phenomena of life occurs without their presence. They are divided into animal proteids and vegetable proteids, between which no essential differences appear. Some chemists use the word albuminoid to mean proteid.

The other forms of the simplest elements of food, the carbohydrates, starches, sugars, fats and mineral matters, are sufficiently explained for our purposes by their very names. Having thus given this discussion of the elements of food, let us now consider how much food is required for the daily use of man. Nature has used these simplest elements in a great variety of forms, the flesh of different animals, in grains, fruits and vegetables, which have different appearances and tastes, and appeal to the appetite in different ways. It remains for man to make the proper use of these food materials.

THE AMOUNT OF FOOD REQUIRED BY MAN.

Scientists have made many analyses of the different foods and many experiments to determine just how much food a person in health ought to have in order to supply the necessary amount of heat and energy to maintain his health and to enable him to do his daily work. One of the scientists, Billings, thinks that an adult male, doing moderate manual labor, ought to eat, every day, twenty ounces of lean meat, twenty-two ounces of bread and ten ounces of potatoes, or the equivalent of these materials in other forms of food, together with three or four cups of coffee. A robust man weighing 144 pounds may consume one-twenty-fourth of his body weight, or six pounds, in nourishment, every day, distributed as follows:

Inorganic food, water and salts, 3.5 pounds, organic food, such as animal food, one pound, vegetable food, one and a half pounds.

Another scientist, Pavy, thinks a man should eat two pounds of bread and three-fourths of a pound of beef, as weighed before it is cooked. This, he thinks, would contain about the right proportion of carbon and nitrogen. This would be forty-four ounces of solid food per day.

The quantity of mineral matter for daily use varies from half an ounce to one ounce. Another scientist estimates that a man of 150 pounds can do an average day's work upon a diet of albuminoids, four and a half ounces; fats, three and three-fourths ounces, carbohydrates, eighteen ounces, and salts, one and one-half ounces. This estimate is for foods free from water.

According to American doctors the quantity of water drank each day is usually less than should be taken. Many persons believe that it is injurious to drink much fluid with their meals, and forget to take it between meals and, as a result, not enough water is consumed to dissolve thoroughly and to eliminate the waste matter from the system. The average quantity of urine voided is fifty-two ounces. Ten ounces are lost from the surface of the lungs and eighteen ounces from the skin. This total loss of eighty ounces must be replaced daily in order to maintain the equilibrium of the body. The solid foods of a mixed diet have been shown to contain on an average, fifty to sixty per cent. of water, so that about twenty-five ounces of water are taken into the system daily as an integral portion of the food. In addition, at least fifty-five ounces or more should be drank, either as plain water or in various beverages. The ratio of solid to liquid foods should be about as one to two.

It is estimated that in each twenty-four hours a man of noraml health and physique absorbs, including the respiratory oxygen and water, about seven and a quarter pounds of material, which he eliminates in a corresponding quantity of waste, about three-fifths of which is water.

THE BEST FOODS TO USE.

Having now given the reader some idea of the amount of food that is required, in a state of health, to maintain health, let us consider for a moment, the best foods that can be used. We shall find that they are principally the foods that we have placed upon our bills of fare for the use of invalids. We are considering, now, the question of food solely from the point of view of health and without reference either to its cost or to satisfying the demands of a more or less capricious palate.

Professor Atwater, whom we have already quoted, has given us the results of experiments with University boat crews, in training for races. These men required the very best foods because they were laboring severely, and were also endeavoring to maintain the best state of health and not only to repair all tissue waste and loss, but to increase their strength and muscular development. We may, therefore, accept the foods that they used as being the best that could be obtained.

We find that the foods that were served to these healthy, well-developed and active young men consisted of roast and broiled beef and lamb, fricassed chicken, roast turkey, broiled fish, eggs, either raw, poached or boiled in the shells, milk and cream, oatmeal, hominy, toasted bread, shredded wheat, cornmeal, bread, potatoes, boiled rice, beets, parsnips, green peas, spinach, asparagus, tomatoes, macaroni, vermicelli, apple tapioca pudding, bread pudding, custard pudding. A small amount of coffee jelly was served, and very rarely, ice cream. No fresh fruit was served with the exception of a few oranges. Stewed prunes, rhubarb and apples were allowed; also dates and figs.

Now there are a few of the above mentioned articles of diet which we should not recommend to invalids, and we should object, as a rule, to some of the methods of cooking. But the reader will see that this diet contains many of the articles which we have placed upon our bills of fare.

A COMPARISON OF FOOD VALUES.

American chemists have analyzed all kinds of food for the purpose of discovering which are the best, the cheapest and the most wholesome. We do not care to give an extended discussion of these results of chemical analysis because that would be out of place here. But we wish to present the analysis of a very few articles which illustrates the points that we have been making in the preceding pages. The analysis shows the protein, the fats, the carbohydrates and the fuel value in each article, and is as follows:

Food	Protein.	Fat.	Carbohydrates.	Mineral Matter.	Fuel Value.
Sirloin of beef	4.25	4.64	.....	0.22	60.62
Milk	1.02	1.13	1.32	0.20	20.31
Butter	0.28	23.48	0.14	0.85	217.18
Salt Pork	1.84	16.88	.....	1.05	164.67
Chicken	3.79	2.88	.....	0.22	42.50
Eggs	4.24	2.97	.....	0.25	44.89
Whole wheat bread	2.45	1.70	18.13	0.85	100.30
Oatmeal	4.42	2.06	19.38	0.53	116.25
Rice	2.20	0.11	22.38	0.11	101.87

The above comparison might be continued indefinitely, but we have stated enough for our purposes. The reader will at once see why milk and rice are wholesome foods in sickness, especially where there is fever. Each of these articles of diet contains all of the elements necessary to support life with a low fuel value. Hence, when a food is desired that will support life and repair the waste of tissue which is a result of disease without creating fever, these two articles are the best to be had. As regards meats we have given the analysis of beer, with much protein and fat and some mineral constituents and a small fuel value and, at the other extreme, salt pork, which contains much less nutriment than beef, but nearly three times as much heat. Hence this latter food would never do for an invalid, or for a well person in a tropical climate. Its use should be confined to healthy, vigorous, hard-working people living in a cold country.

Undoubtedly, the four articles of food that are of the greatest value to the human race are wheat, beef, milk and rice. These are the mainstays of life among the densest populations the world over.

According to this analysis chicken ought also to be a very desirable food in cases of sickness, but there is some quality about this food, not revealed in the analysis, which makes it too strong in critical cases, and we much prefer beef until after our patrons have recovered from the severest attacks and their digestive powers are stronger.

THE FOODS OF THE FUTURE.

After all, considering the length of time that man has been upon the earth, the variety of foods now used by him is less than might be expected, and great numbers of the articles in use are not entirely desirable from the standpoint of health. Realizing this, efforts are constantly being made by some of the leading governments to add new kinds of food, especially grains and vegetables, to those now commonly used. The government of the United States has been active in this direction, and has turned its attention to a considerable extent to that vast empire of China, from which have already come many of the best foods of man, in the hope of discovering there other new varieties of value.

Upon this point Mr. Arthur Henry, in an article entitled "The Foods of the Future," published in the Puritan Magazine for November, 1899, has the following to say:

"A dozen plants will cover the vegetable display on the average American table from one year's end to another. If the experiments recently undertaken by the Agricultural Department prove successful, the dozen will be multiplied by hundreds. A government food expert has recently estimated that the number of vegetables, all of which could be grown for the table, would reach into hundreds.

"Onions, horseradish, cucumbers and melons all originated wild in the Orient. Fifty years ago England sent out the explorer Fortune, who brought back with him a rémarkable collection of plants which made him famous. Among these was the Chinese sand pear, in itself a purely ornamental species, bearing fruit that is scarcely edible, and yet from which, by a process of culture, resulted the Kieffer and Le Conte varieties, which have revolutionized pear culture in the southern part of the United States.

"It has been estimated by Mr. Augustine Henry, well known for his researches on the Chinese flora, that there are at least one hundred kinds of fruits growing wild and unknown in the interior of

China which could be cultivated and made as valuable to the use of man as either the peach or the apple."

NEW FOODS FROM CHINA.

Walter C. Blasdale, instructor in chemistry in the University of California, another expert for the United States Government, has recently rendered a report on certain Chinese vegetable food materials, of which he has made an exhaustive study. He believes that many of these will ultimately become of general use and of great value to American and European nations. Among the plants which he discusses are the saggitaria, or arrowhead which produces tubers "of about the same consistency as a potato, yellowish in color and farinaceous in taste," the taro, which has furnished food from remote antiquity to the natives of southern India, Australia, portions of Africa, and many of the islands of the Pacific, and is today one of the plants most commonly cultivated throughout the tropics; the water chestnut, which is a very valuable plant and has medicinal qualities not yet understood by Mr. Blasdale, but of great importance. Mr. Blasdale considers them a very palatable article of food. He also speaks of the sacred lotus of which, among other things, he says: "The seeds contain a white starch used largely as food; roasted and ground they served the Egyptians for the manufacture of a kind of bread; in China they are used in soup and also as a remedy for indigestion. They are supposed to have invigorative properties when used as food by convalescents. The Chinese also extract from the root a starch which they say is very strengthening."

This writer also discusses the value as food of the Chinese sweet potatoes, the yam beans, the cassava or manioc, several varieties of green vegetables, used in China but little known in this country or in Europe; soy beans and several other varieties of similar vegetables, and several kinds of fruits, nuts and edible flowers. He considers that many of these might prove of great value in America if they were properly cultivated and if a thorough test were given of their merits.

This report is valuable as showing the interest of the great American people in the products of the vast and ancient Chinese

Empire, and also as showing the demand for new foods and the importance attached to all products of the vegetable kingdom that are available for the use of man. The Chinese have used these foods and plants, and thousands of others, from the very beginning of their history, and have, from their long experience, developed not only a system of diet, but a system of purely herbal medication which have been of great importance in making the immense population of China hardy and long-lived.

CHAPTER III.

INFORMATION FOR PATRONS AND INQUIRERS.

Suggestions as to the Points of Difference Between This System and Others—How the Treatment Should Be Commenced and Continued.

For the Special Benefit of Chronic Sufferers.

The following remarks and instructions should be carefully read and observed by all persons who desire benefit from our treatment. This system of medication is different from any other, and its efficacy depends upon certain simple and logical principles. If these are fully understood and carefully followed, the benefit received in any case will be greatly increased. In fact, such observance is essential to satisfactory results.

We do not make the absurd claim advanced by many physicians, or at least indicated in their lack of attention to diet and simple laws of health, that medicines will work miracles. Medicines properly used assist nature in her constant effort to throw off disease. It is natural for people to be well. But medicines cannot make them well if they oppose the processes of cure, by late hours, narcotic, over-eating, dissipation in any form, or other practices that tend to lower vitality and hinder recuperation from the effects of disease.

The first essential is attention to diet, which should be restricted. We prescribe a dietary for each patient which should in all cases be strictly followed. When a person's system is clogged with impurities and the vital organs are hindered in their functions, a large amount of food cannot be assimilated. It is simply so much more foreign matter which must be thrown off before the vital organs can resume their customary duties. It not only does no good, but is in the way, and therefore does actual harm. Furthermore, the remedies which we prescribe are in themselves foods and in a large measure take the place of other articles of diet. For this reason the patient requires less food than he would need were he not taking treatment.

These remedies frequently cause patients pain, and dull, ill-defined uneasiness for periods varying with the different conditions of different cases. These indications that the medicines are working in the system should cause no alarm. They are simply proofs that nature is ridding the system of the obnoxious elements which oppose a cure. Sometimes the pain is felt in the head, resulting in headache and giddiness. In other cases the symptoms take the form of frequent and sometimes violent purgings. Sometimes there is simply a sensation of lassitude and aversion to the ordinary duties of life. To be forewarned is to be forearmed, and our patrons are hereby advised of the fact that these circumstances are not unfavorable. On the contrary they indicate that the remedies are producing the desired effect. They will gradually wear away and will be followed by a reaction which will finally result in increased energy and a restoration of health. Our medicines are neither tonics nor purgatives. They are simply assistants to the vital organs in a resumption of their proper duties. Purging is an effort of nature to rid itself of obnoxious elements and not a direct result of the medicines.

Persons desiring relief from chronic diseases must have patience to continue the treatment. An impaired constitution cannot be restored in a day, and the remedial processes of nature are always slow.

Many persons show a childishly thoughtless anxiety to be cured at once. They forget that a demoralized body, which has been gradually deteriorating for months or years, cannot be restored to its normal condition in a few days, or, in some instances, even in a few weeks. They fail to comprehend that the system must frequently be cleansed of a load of impurities and debris, the result of impaired nutrition, poisonous and mineral medication, imperfect circulation and other derangements of the bodily powers, before a cure can be commenced. They want to discover a substantial improvement at once. We do not promise such improvement. We cannot accomplish what nature never undertakes to do. A tree which has been nearly killed by drought may sometimes be restored to health by care, irrigation and cultivation; but it does not bear fruit the second week after it is watered. It first puts out its new buds upon the lower branches and afterwards upon those more distant from the roots, showing a gradual re-establishment of a circulation of the tree's life juices. In due time the leaves follow, then the flowers and finally the fruit. The restoration of a crippled and degenerate body, whose functions are abnormal, is a somewhat similar process, and depends upon laws which are as invariable as the laws of growth in the vegetable kingdom. Do not expect impossibilities and you will not be disappointed. Any physician who guarantees cures of chronic ailments in a brief period of time simply plays upon the credulity of his patients and soothes their aches and pains by powerful narcotics into a deceptive condition of apparent but unreal improvement. Diet, regimen and careful and continued medication are essential factors in any genuine and lasting benefit

Bear in mind that what appears to be self-denial in obeying the rules is really an earnest effort on the part of the patient to help himself. It is a part of the treatment—co-operation—which is solely for the patient's benefit and depends entirely upon his powers of will. Excessive sexual or other indulgence is always to be avoided. No medicines in the world will build up an impoverished body if it's already exhausted vitality is still constantly drawn upon. Common sense and a little reflection on the part of the patient will show him at once the reasonableness of these facts. Three, six, or even nine months is a very short period in the life of a man, and if self-denial and strict regard for a hygienic regimen during that time will restore a sick man to the priceless boon of health, which the united wealth of the world alone could not buy, the self-sacrifice involved is certainly abundantly rewarded.

CAUTION TO PATIENTS.

The Chinese system of medicine avoids the use of both tonics and purgatives. The remedies employed are not designed to give a fictitious and temporary renewal of strength to a worn-out frame. Nor are they used to work sudden and violent effects such as follows the use of calomel and similar purgatives. Purging, when it follows the employment of these remedies, is simply the elimination of impurities preceding a gradual restoration of normal conditions. The value of diet is recognized emphatically and patients are usually placed upon a plain and simple bill of fare, which, while sufficient for the maintenance of strength, is yet such as to reduce inflammation and to assist the remedies in their beneficial effects upon the stomach and other organs. These remedies are in themselves special foods, and the patient requires less of his ordinary meat and drink while taking them. Lack of care in this respect results in overloading the stomach and defeating the proper action of the remedies. Great care must also be used to avoid exposure to cold while using them.

These restrictions, together with certain phenomena which frequently attend the use of these remedies, are so different from the "painless dentistry" methods of some physicians that patients often become discouraged. They are sometimes troubled with a slight nausea, with dizziness, with ill-defined feelings of uneasiness or with actual pains in different parts of the body. These manifestations are simply indications that the remedies are performing their customary and proper work. But it is frequently difficult for the patient to believe this fact, which is at variance with his prejudices and preconceived notions of the objects of medical treatment. He sometimes becomes discouraged after a few weeks and discontinues the treatment just when he should cling most closely to it. As a rule, the alarming indications pass away in a few days. In many cases they do not occur at all. Yet some of our best friends today are persons who became discouraged and withdrew from treatment after following it for a short time. Fortunately, sufficient had been accomplished to have a decidedly beneficial effect after the system had had time to resume what may be called a condition of equilibrium. With an improvement in health many of these persons have seen their mistake and resumed treatment, but with loss of time and of the cumulative force of the remedies, and consequently with an increased ultimate expense.

We prefer to be perfectly frank with our patients, and we desire that these facts should be fully understood. We recognize that persons in ill-health are entitled to a little consideration such as we would not expect to accord to people in good health. And we find that men, as a rule, are more capricious than women, and less capable of enduring aches, pains and restrictions necessary to recovery. Of all classes active business men are the most difficult to convince of the necessity of care and rest when sensations of illness are commencing to grow upon them. They think they cannot afford the time necessary for a cure, and they are so irregular in respect to their meals and in taking of the remedies that cures are very greatly hindered, if not rendered impossible. For these reasons we are thus particular in making these explanations. We recognize the limitations of all medical systems, and know that medicines will not work miracles. We desire to warn our patients against probable discouragements and prefer to state the facts ourselves rather than to have them stated, with exaggerations, by some person who feels himself aggrieved because we have not performed more than was promised. These remarks apply particularly to cases of long standing, or very severe diseases. In acute attacks and those of recent origin, a great benefit is often derived within a very few days.

SOME POINTS TO BE OBSERVED.

Avoid excitement of every character, cast aside all anxiety and make earnest and persistent efforts to assist nature to restore the deranged condition of the system by preserving the vital forces in every manner possible.

Do not chew gum or toothpicks, or anything that will cause saliva to flow between meal hours. Such practices are very weakening to the system, causing thirst and a weak, scant supply of juices in the stomach and bowels.

Avoid large gatherings in crowded halls or apartments. The inhaling of the foul air at such places, together with the exposure at a late hour at night, is a practice that is very injurious to the health of even robust people.

Hold in check all desires that if indulged in will tend to weaken the system. A candle will last only half as long a time if allowed to burn at both ends as it will if there is a fire at only one end. The same reason applies to human life.

Without proper nutrition there could be but little or no benefit derived by taking medicine.

Retire regularly at an early hour. One hour's sleep before midnight is worth more to a young growing, laboring or sick person than two hours after.

Do not occupy a bed with another. You need all of the pure air you can get, and should live as quiet a life as possible. Take as much sleep as you feel like.

Married people should bear in mind that certain indulgences which may be perfectly proper when in health are decidedly injurious when persons are ill or weakly. Entire abstinence is the best rule for a time, especially when either the husband or wife is commencing a course of treatment.

Invalids should wear flannel all the year round, and during the winter season the warmest that can be procured.

With people who are in poor health, bodily heat should be husbanded in every possible way. The degree of warmth and comfort that a weakly person enjoys depends greatly upon the quality of the material of which the clothing is made.

Be very particular to avoid exposure to draughts of air just after taking the herb teas, or having taken a meal. If at such times you perspire or feel at all uncomfortably warm, you should wipe the perspiration off as much of the body as you can conveniently, and then bring the clothing about the body so as to protect it from the cool air, for a short time at least. Many weakly people recklessly expose themselves by throwing open their dwellings as soon as they feel a little uncomfortably warm.

In warm weather, when you perspire freely, you should change underwear often to prevent the perspiration from returning to the skin, which is very serious to the health. It is equal to taking so much poison.

In very warm weather the skin should be rubbed two or three times daily with a warm, wet towel, to remove the perspiration.

BATHING AND RUBBING.

You should take a warm sponge bath as follows: Bathe the lower half of the body one day, and the upper portion three or four days later. The bath always to be warm and of short duration, so as not to take cold; use one-half cup of alcohol in hot water. In the season of the year when you perspire more or less, a sponge bath may be indulged in every other day. Invalids in all stages of disease, and also well persons, should brush or rub (with a flesh brush or warm towel) the body moderately. This practice is very essential and beneficial to health, and should be practiced daily, but not to the extent that will cause fatigue.

When the body is exposed to the cold air with which it comes in contact when the clothing is removed to take a bath or to retire or for any other purpose, it allows the bodily heat to escape, which is a loss of power and lowers the temperature of the skin, taxing the powers of the system to warm up the new air to protect the body. The air surrounding the body is the armor of the body. If the air is strong in the body (and a strong person possesses strong air) the person will not be injured by bathing; but a weakly person will, soon after taking a bath, have a weak and heavy feeling, which is evidence that the skin has taken on damp air and has lost control of the natural air The air in a weak person is like a small capital that is depended upon to accomplish a given purpose—it must be handled with care and to the very best advantage, or else the capital and object will both be lost, and perhaps a good cause forever buried.

Hand rubbing, if performed properly, would be very beneficial to nearly every weakly person. The full size of the shoulder and chest should be (each side) rubbed toward and down the arms to the end of the fingers; from the shoulders and the chest rub downwards and to the ends of the toes. The rubbing should be proceeded with slowly, extending over only a small surface at first, then extending over additional surface, commencing at the starting point with each pressure of the hands on the patient. Commence with one rubbing a day, not less than two hours after a meal, to be completed in twenty minutes; two or three rubbings may be practiced a day, as the strength improves. If you feel like it, take undisturbed rest or sleep after the rubbing, but be particular to guard against taking cold. No matter how comfortably warm you feel, fully as much or more covering to the body is necessary after the rubbing as before, especially if the patient lie down

BREATHING EXERCISE.

Renovate the system in the morning after the sun is up in the following manner: If you are unable to ride on horseback or to walk fast enough to cause rapid breathing, the foul air may be expelled from the system while standing in the sunlight and breathing deep and fast enough to work the abdomen vigorously, taking from three to five breaths in rapid succession; then resting a few minutes until the dizziness which usually follows with weakly persons passes away, then repeat several times, always breathing through the nostrils.

Spend as much time as possible in the open air and sunshine, and while walking about make a practice of taking long, deep breaths.

These exercises are very beneficial to the lungs and stimulating to the whole system. Air is an indispensable element, and artfully used is a wonderful agent in purifying the human system; the long, deep breaths taken in slowly and held while taking five to ten steps, allowing the weight of the body to rest on the heel of one foot rather heavily, sufficient to jar the body to some extent, which will tend to force the stale and impure air or gases out of the system. These gases are always present in systems that are weakly, the practice must be indulged in with great care and moderation, or else much harm will result; therefore increase the frequency of deep inhalations slowly as time goes on, until the number of forty or fifty a day is reached. You should be out in the open air on bright, warm, sunny days, but avoid taking these exercises and being out of doors in damp or cold weather; at such times take the exercise in the house.

FRESH AIR IN SLEEPING ROOMS.

Always have plenty of fresh air in your sleeping room. This should be managed so that you will not be affected by draughts, but the air should always be fresh and pure. Many people are so afraid of taking cold that they close their windows tightly at night, with the result that they breathe the same air over and over during the night. This is a very serious mistake and prevents many people from recovering. Even consumptives who come to Southern California for the benefit of the fresh, pure, out-door air, close their windows and breathe the same poisonous atmosphere again and again. It is no wonder that so many of them fail to regain their health. This is a very important point, for pure air, which means an abundance of oxygen, is more important to weak and ill people than an abundance of food even. Its value cannot be over estimated.

BE ON YOUR GUARD AGAINST COLDS.

Sitting or lying in draughts or currents of air is something that is very necessary for invalids to guard against, as such exposure will in a short time cause you to take cold. You would be less exposed and better off out of doors in the open air, on bright, sunny days, than sitting in a draught, as stated.

While you were in perfect health, your circulation good, such exposure would have no bad effects upon you; but you must not forget that you are an invalid now, that the "door is open" as it were, and you are more susceptible to colds. Of all the accidents that our patients are liable to encounter, colds are far the worst, and are really to be dreaded; very often a simple cold causes the worst form of sickness, and also death.

Some patients feel quite languid or weak after taking the medicines awhile, for a short time, which is the result of the medicines searching the system and also allaying the inflammation which is present in nearly all cases of ill-health. Inflammation is strength for a time, or as long as the powers will endure that condition. Some people exercise so much strength while in a fever that the combined strength of two or three men is required to keep the patient on the bed and to prevent him from doing himself harm; but when the inflammation subsides a very weak condition follows. We do not produce a sudden change in such conditions—we reduce the inflammation slowly; it is the only way to effect a cure in cases of long standing—sudden changes often produce disastrous results.

When you feel drowsy, or as if you didn't care to move about or eat or talk (such feelings will appear frequently as long as the impurities remain in your system), make it a practice to keep quiet for a day or two, till the condition changes, and allow the medicine to carry out its work; you will sooner arrive at a condition of better feelings than you would if you allowed yourself to worry and get excited because you were feeling worse than when you commenced the treatment. Your feelings are not a correct index to the condition of your system, neither can you predict the condition that you will be in on the morrow.

SOME HANDY REMEDIES.

The following simple prescriptions are given herewith for the benefit of all and to meet the emergencies which are likely to arise any day and in any household. They do not cost much, yet may be of great value:

No. 1—For Skin Diseases and Rheumatic Pains in the Limbs or Feet.

Take orange leaves, one-fourth pound,
Honeysuckle leaves or flowers (the latter are best) two ounces.
Black tea, one ounce.

The orange and honeysuckle leaves must be washed until clean. Put all into seven cupfuls of water and boil for half an hour. Use as a wash upon the parts affected. If a larger quantity is desired two or three cups of boiling water may be added, or if it desired to be kept hot a long time, the same amount of boiling water may be added for this purpose. It is always to be applied hot, as the heat gives more benefit from the wash.

Persons who are using herbs for internal use in cases of rheumatism or skin diseases can take the refuse of the herbs after they have been cooked for the internal use. Add the orange leaves as above. If honeysuckle leaves or flowers are easy to get, add those also, but leave out the black tea. Put in the water as indicated and boil as directed above. This also makes an excellent wash for these diseases. Always use it hot.

No. 2—To Quench Thirst.

Take four dried figs and three cupfuls of water and boil down to two cups. The liquid resulting makes a pleasant and healthful drink. Some people like it for food also. If a larger quantity is desired, double the number of figs and the amount of water.

No. 3—Remedy for Constipation.

Into two cupfuls of water put four tablespoonfuls of strained honey. Stir the mixture and use as an injection. The water must be warm. This injection, from the soothing qualities of the honey, will remove inflammation from the bowels and does not hurt the natural juices upon which the healthy action of the bowels depend. If the bowels do not move, repeat the injection the next day in the following manner: Take two ounces of Maderia vine and clean it thoroughly. Add three cups of water and boil down to two. Add honey the same as before and use as an injection. The addition of the Maderia vine makes the prescription stronger than before.

Whenever cups are mentioned in these prescriptions, large coffee cups are intended.

No. 4—A Cure for Stomach Ache.

Take half a cup of salt and heat it by stirring it in a hot pan. Put the hot salt in a handkerchief or similar cloth and wrap it up. Then gently pat and rub the skin over the part where the ache is. This will relieve the pain by quickening the circulation and by warming the stomach and the blood. This method will also relieve pains in the bones and any part of the body. It will be found useful for pains in the back.

No. 5—Treatment of Burns and Scaldings.

For a burn or scalding on the hands or fingers do not put the injured part in the water—a process which is the natural proceeding with many people. If the part is put into cold water the fire poison will go deeper and will return inside. Sometimes it will go very deep and cause a great deal of pain and trouble. Instead of water dip the finger or hand into kerosene oil and the fire poison will return to the skin. Keep the injured part out of water for two or three days. If there is a very great injury, consult Drs. Foo and Wing as soon as possible, but the oil will relieve for a time.

No. 6—Wash for the Eye.

Chrysanthemum flowers steeped in water make a good wash for the eye. Take one cup and a half of water and one or two ounces of the flowers. Boil down to one cup. The white variety of the flowers is the best. This will afford temporary relief for sore eyes until our remedies may be used to remove the cause of the difficulty from the inside of the body. Steaming the eyes is also good, but if this is done care must be taken to steam both eyes, even though it is supposed that only one is affected, because when the eyes are steamed the poisonous matter which results from inflammation, will go from one to the other. This method will relieve the symptoms, but it is better to take the herb medicines and to remove the cause of the difficulty from the vital organs.

EASY BUT USEFUL EXERCISES.

No. 1—To Exercise the Nerves and Pulse of the Body.

Stand erect, clench the fists and draw them up to the sides of the upper chest, with the elbows drawn well back; then raise the arms straight up from the shoulders, three times and back; putting vitality in them, as if you were raising a weight, with the eyes looking straight down the nose.

No. 2.

Take the same position as before, then raise one arm at a time alternately, three times each; going through the same movement as No. 1.

No. 3—To Exercise the Chest and Back-bone.

Stand erect, extend the arms in the same direction, first to the right and then to the left.

No. 4—To Exercise the Heart.

Stand erect and perfectly still, turn the head to the right as far as possible, holding it about five seconds, then turn it back straight and belch—or attempt to—repeat this six or seven times; after which turn the head to the left, going through the same movement. This exercise causes the heart to expand, and moves the foul air, making the circulation strong.

No. 5—To Exercise the Eyes.

Close the fists and raise them to the temples, near the eyes, and extend them at full length, in front of the body and back, at the same time keeping the eyes on an object directly in front of you.

No. 6—To Exercise the Stomach and Assist Digestion.

Close the fists and draw them up near the shoulders, take a few steps to the right, then to the left, then stop and stand with the feet about three feet apart, stooping over slightly (as if riding horseback) and remain in that position as long as you can, or until you feel exhausted.

No. 7—To Exercise the Lower Extremities and the Stomach.

Clasp the hands behind you, and walk for a few minutes at a brisk pace, bringing the feet down hard upon the ground.

No. 8—To Exercise the Nerves.

Extend the arms in front of you, lower them and touch (or attempt to touch) the toes, without bending the knees. Repeat this three or four times.

No. 9—Exercise for the Lungs.

Stand erect in the open air or in a well ventilated room, inhale and exhale full short breaths for one or two minutes, working the chest vigorously; after which take a full breath through the mouth and hold it a little while, walking twenty or thirty steps, and striking the feet hard upon the ground or floor.

No. 10—To Exercise the Liver and Make the Blood Circulate Freely.

Close the eyes and roll them sidewise, right and left, for one or two minutes. This exercise is also beneficial to the eyes, making the vision clearer; as the eyes are connected with the liver by hollow nerves, which the air circulates between.

No. 11—Exercise for the Brain.

Place the palms of the hands over the ears, closing the drums completely, and drum on the head with the fingers for one or two minutes; this tends to remove the foul air from the head and quiets the mind. Laboring men and those engaged in business should practice this morning and evening, and people of leisure three times a day.

No. 12—Exercise for the Stomach.

Soon after eating a meal take the following exercise: While walking slowly, place the palm of the hand upon the abdomen and rub, medium hard, over the spleen and around the stomach for a few minutes. This will assist the spleen and digestive organs to perform their functions.

No. 13—Exercise for the Back.

Stand erect, and cross the arms in front, placing the hands upon the shoulders, then turn the upper portion of the body from side to side, as far as possible without moving the lower portion of the body. Repeat several times.

FOO & WING HERB COMPANY

> CHINESE CONSULATE GENERAL
> SAN FRANCISCO
>
> December 17th 1899.
>
> To whom it may concern:
>
> I beg to certify that the bearer, whose photograph is hereunder attached, is Tom Foo Yuen, a member of the Imperial College of Medicine in Pekin and a graduate thereof.
>
> He has had many year's experience in China and has achieved a deserved reputation as a Physician.
>
> Ho Yow, 何祐
> H. I. C. M's Consul General.
>
> This photo is the true likeness of the above named Tam Foo Yuen.

The above is a fac-simile of a new certificate recently issued to Tom Foo Yuen by Ho Yow, the present Consul-General of the Chinese government at San Francisco.

CHAPTER IV.

Tom Foo Yuen—Some Account of This Oriental Physician—His Diplomas and Credentials—A Brief History of His Life and Experiences in America.

In the following pages is a brief statement of Tom Foo Yuen's career in the United States. But before giving this we shall present some of his diplomas and other credentials, showing his rank in China and the high esteem in which he is held by men of exalted position in his own country. We give a fac-simile and a translation of his first diploma, received from the Imperial Medical College at Peking. The original of this document is a sheet of satin, royal gold in color, so called from the fact that it is used in China only by the Emperor, and for state documents. The diploma is printed upon this in red letters. Accompanying is a fac-simile of the Chinese original:

Following is the English translation of this diploma:

JOYOUS ANNOUNCEMENT.

His Majesty, the Emperor, has appointed His Excellency, the Honorable Fook, Chief Guardian of His Royal Highness, the Prince Heir Apparent, President of the Board of Population and Revenue, Member of the Privy Council, Dean of the Imperial Medical College, and Blood Relative to His Majesty, His Excellency, the Honorable Chung, Assistant Magistrate of the Left Chamber in the Imperial Medical College, Mandarin of the Second Degree of the Order of the Peacock Feather.

His Excellency, the Honorable Lee, Assistant Magistrate of the Right Chamber in the Imperial Medical College, Mandarin of the Second Degree of the Order of the Peacock Feather, as His Majesty's

FOO & WING HERB COMPANY

WITH THE SEAL OF ROYALTY

Translation and Explanation of T. Foo Yuen's Royal Gold Diploma, Fac-simile of a Rare and Interesting Document, the First Authentic One of its Kind Ever Presented to the English Speaking People. Its Owner the First Physician of His Rank and Scholarship to Come to America.

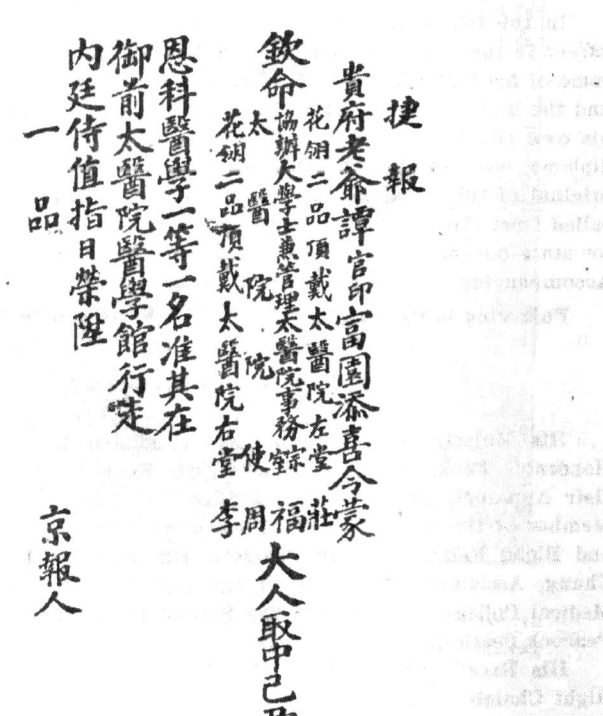

Imperial Deputation, to conduct the Special Grace Examination in the Imperial Medical College, who have conferred upon Tom Foo Yuen a First Rank of the First Degree in the Year Ki Chen of Cyclical Table, or in the 15th year of the Reign of Kong Sui. (1889).

And therefore, they, clothed with such authority, have passed Tom Foo Yuen, a member of Your Worthy Family, with highest honors, and have conferred upon him the right to practice before His Majesty and in the Imperial Medical College.

May good fortune abide with him upon his way to the highest degree.

Some explanation of the peculiar wording of a portion of the above may perhaps be necessary. It is customary in China when a student passes difficult examinations mentioned, to send a messenger to his family bearing the good news. On the return of this messenger the document is published in the principal newspapers of the capital and of other cities of the empire as an act of courtesy to the sovereign. The diploma is here given just as it originally appeared in the Post Courier, published in Pekin.

After receiving the diploma, Tom Foo Yuen was entitled and permitted to undertake a second examination for still further honors. It may be said in explanation that there were 487 members of this class, of whom Tom Foo Yuen was adjudged to be the first by his mark of standing in the different studies of the course. Only seven of the nearly five hundred members of this class succeeded in passing the difficult examinations which entitled them to the diploma already given. These seven were then given a second examination to determine whether they were worthy of a second and greater honor. Four of the seven succeeded in passing this second examination. Tom Foo Yuen standing highest of the four, and these were awarded a second diploma, a translation of which we give herewith. This second diploma entitles the holder, after a lapse of twelve years, to a position as instructor in the Imperial Medical College, and the right to practice in the family of His Majesty, the Emperor of China. During the intervening twelve years the candidate is presumed to perfect himself for such instruction and practice by the active employment of his talents and acquirements as a physician. At the end of that period he presents himself at the college and is invested with the titles, dignities and emoluments of an instructor. It will readily be seen that this is an honor for which thousands would willingly labor diligently for a lifetime.

FOLLOWING IS A TRANSLATION OF THE SECOND DIPLOMA.

By Imperial Decree the following were named as His Majesty's deputation to select and detain at the Medical College for Imperial employment the most skillful of the successful candidates at the Grace Examination at Peking, which gathered from the different provinces of the Empire in the year Ki Chew of Cyclical Tables.

His Excellency, the Honorable Fook, Blood Relative to His Majesty, Member of the Privy Council, President of the Imperial Medical College; His Excellency, the Honorable Chow, High Imperial Commissioner of the Imperial Medical College; His Excellency, the Honorable Chung, Mandarin of the Second Degree of the Order of the Peacock Feather, Director of the Left Chamber of the Imperial Medical College; and His Excellency, the Honorable Lee, Mandarin of the Second Degree of the Order of the Peacock Feather, Director of the Right Chamber of the Imperial Medical College.

And, therefore, in the exercise of their authority, granted for this purpose, they have selected Tom Foo Yuen, of the District of Shuen Tak, Province of Kwang Tung, head of the highest class of the medical candidates, profoundly skillful in the principle of the pulse, and thoroughly versed in the nature of medicine, and have caused his name to be registered in the official record Of which action this is a certificate, and the same is to be delivered to Tom Foo Yuen, of the Imperial Medical College of Peking.

Kwung-Sui, 15th year, ninth month and the 20th day (1889).

(Official Seal).

FOO & WING HERB COMPANY

The following certificate was given to Tom Foo Yuen by the Chinese Consul General, formerly resident of San Francisco, on his first coming to California:

CERTIFICATE.

Office 806 Stockton Street,
Imperial Chinese Consulate General,
San Francisco, 24th March, 1893.

This is to certify that I, Li Yung Yew, His Imperial Majesty's Consul General to the Port of San Francisco, have known Tom Foo Yuen for many years; I know him to have been a member of Imperial College of Medicine in Peking, and to be a graduate thereof; that he has for several years practiced his profession in China, and that he has there achieved marked success as a physician.

(LI YUNG YEW)

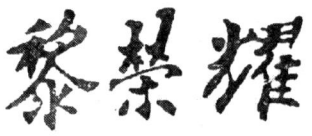

[SEAL]

H. I. C. M.'s Consul General.

BIOGRAPHICAL SKETCH OF TOM FOO YUEN.

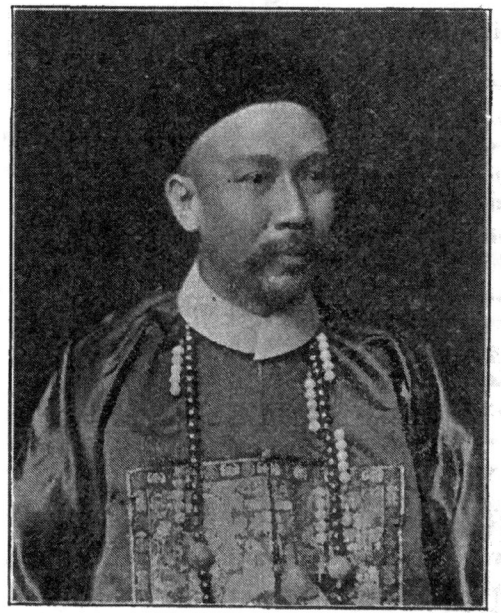

Tom Foo Yuen was born near Canton, China, in 1855, and was educated at the Imperial Medical College at Peking. When he was only a little boy he made a trip to San Francisco with his father, and resided there for a short time. His father was a wealthy physician—the late Dr. T. Gee Son—and was also engaged in mercantile ventures as the president of a great mercantile association. In a general way he superintended the legal and business affairs of his company, and was on business of this sort when he brought his little son to America. Tom Foo Yuen's mother was a sister of the celebrated Chinese physician, Dr. Li Po Tai.

About thirty years ago Dr. T. Gee Son lived in San Francisco for several years as a partner of Li Po Tai. Together they cured the diseases of many Americans, and testimonials of these cures were printed in the newspapers of the period. But his family preferred the climate of Canton to that of San Francisco, and they therefore returned to Canton, where T. Gee Son again opened a hospital that he had formerly conducted with great success.

Returning to China with his father, Tom Foo Yuen was educated as a physician with all the care and rigorous discipline usual in China, where successive generations are trained for this profession from the commencement of school days. He was finally graduated, with high honors, from the Imperial Medical College at Peking. In 1890 he came to San Francisco and was the first Oriental physician of his rank to visit America with the intention of making a permanent home here. He became an associate with Li Po Tai, who was then getting old and unable to carry on all of his large business.

He remained in San Francisco until 1893 and, during that time acquired an enviable reputation as a physician, both among the Chinese residents of San Francisco and among many white patrons.

He was very successful in all cases. Of late years, since Tom Foo Yuen commenced to attain his great popularity in Southern California, it has been the fashion in some quarters, among those who envy his accomplishments, to attempt to underrate his ability; and statements have been made that he is not a graduate of the Imperial Medical College at Peking. He has many diplomas and certificates which set this question fully at rest. Among the proofs of the genuineness of his claims is one not heretofore published. The Chinese patients whom he cured in San Francisco were not likely to be deceived in reference to his merits and attainments, as they had every opportunity to investigate and verify his claims. Many of these gave him testimonials of the cures that he wrought in their cases, and two of these testimonials, which were printed in Chinese newspapers, published in San Francisco, are reproduced herewith to show that he was recognized by his own countrymen, at the outset of his career, as a man of the most thorough education and the most eminent qualifications in his profession.

The first of these is from the Weekly Occident, published by Horn, Hong & Co., at 731 Washington street, San Francisco. Vol. 12. No. 615, February 23, 1893. We give it in both English and Chinese. It says:

"After years of suffering and having been under the treatment of some of the most skillful Chinese and American doctors, I placed myself under the care of Dr. Tom Foo Yuen, who is a graduate of the Imperial Medical College at Peking. I take pleasure in testifying to the fact of his having effected a complete cure of what was pronounced by others a hopeless case of consumption. Chow Yup Wing.

"The doctor's office is at No. 729 Washington street."

The second of these testimonials is from the Weekly News, Mon Heng & Co., publishers, 809½ Washington street, San Francisco, Vol. 1, No. 4, Thursday, February 23, 1893, and reads as follows:

"I have been suffering greatly with paralysis, and I am greatly indebted to Dr. Tom Foo Yuen, a graduate of the Imperial Chinese Medical College at Peking, who has entirely cured me. I desire to make this known to all who may be afflicted with the same disease in order that they may secure his services and be relieved of their suffering. Lum Chuen."

In 1893 Tom Foo Yuen came to Southern California in company with Mr. Levi Carter of Ceres, California, who went to San Francisco to accompany him to Southern California. He came to the southern part of the state partly for the climate, which is more congenial to him than that of San Francisco, and partly to form a partnership in an herb company with an American who had become acquainted with him in San Francisco. For this purpose he went to Redlands, where he remained two years and three months. During the first year of his residence in that city he became much attached to Southern California for its delightful climate and other advantages as a residence, and was very successful in a business way. He cured a great many people in and about Redlands, most of whom had been abandoned by other physicians, whom they had consulted, but who had failed to cure them. Naturally these cures made a great deal of stir in that quiet city, as they were the first evidences which the good people of Redlands had ever seen of merit in the Chinese System of Medicine. Those who beheld the unquestionable results of Foo's methods were greatly astonished, and those who were cured of painful and sometimes threatening diseases, many of which had been pronounced incurable, were naturally very much pleased, and were inclined to tell others about their good fortune. They praised Tom Foo Yuen in the very highest terms, and thus brought about the first of a series of controversies with other physicians, in each of which, as may be remarked in passing, Foo emerged with flying colors. A physician in Redlands became offended at the comparisons made between his own system of practice and that of the Chinese doctor, and attacked Foo and his methods in the Redlands Citrograph. A reporter of the Leader, a rival paper, thereupon interviewed a number of Tom Foo Yuen's patients, and was surprised to learn that they not only freely acknowledged the circumstances of the cures in their cases, but warmly defended him from the extravagant and often abusive charges brought against him by professional rivals. This was a beginning of an open acknowledgment by many persons who have been benefited by his skill as a physician; of the great merit of the system of herbal treatment which he practices. Three of these testimonials given on this occasion were as follows:

Mr. H. W. Timmons of Redlands, being interviewed, said: "For the past two months I have been treated by Dr. Foo for facial rheumatism. I consulted several physicians in Los Angeles and Redlands, but they all admitted they could not cure me. I finally went to Dr. Foo, who after feeling my pulse located my disease. I am now on the road to a speedy recovery." Mrs. Throckmorton, who resides on Church street, Redlands, said: "I think Dr. Foo a man of culture and science, and place every confidence in him. I am a native of New York, where for many years I was a sufferer from chronic bronchitis. I spent thousands of dollars for treatment by all modern physicians, but never received any practical benefit from them. I consulted the very best specialists in the East but they were unable to effect a cure, and advised me to seek a change of climate. I came to Southern California and located here in Redlands. I was advised to consult Dr. Foo. Before doing so, my sister who is a graduate of an Eastern medical college, first went to the doctor to investigate his methods of treatment. The result of her investigations was very satisfactory, so that I went myself to the doctor's office, where he examined me and correctly diagnosed my case by merely feeling the pulse. Since then I have been under Dr. Foo's treatment, and am rapidly recovering renewed health. I have every confidence that Dr. Foo will effect a permanent cure." Dr. B. F. Watrous was next seen at his residence. When asked to give his opinion of Tom Foo Yuen, he said: "I have a very high opinion of Dr. Foo. To him I owe my life. When other physicians failed to cure me, Dr. Foo made a well man of me. I think the article in the Citrograph a cowardly and unwarrantable attack upon Dr. Foo, who, in my opinion, has no equal in this country."

Among others who gave testimonials in Foo's favor on this occasion were Mrs. George Robotham of Newark, N. J.; W. A. Hallowell, Jr., of Ontario; George W. Hazard of Riverside; Mrs. M. H. Wilson, Mrs. Mattie Reeder, Mrs. A. J. Hendrickson, Earl Garrison, Mrs. C. A Kingsbury, G. E. Foster, John McIntosh of Redlands, and Robert McPherson of McPherson, Orange county, Cal. Many of these ladies and gentlemen have continued to be among his best friends and most ardent supporters from that day to the present time.

After the publication of the Leader's answer to the Citrograph nothing more was heard from Dr. Foo's antagonist among the physicians of Redlands, and the excitement subsided. But many people have begun to go to Redlands from Los Angeles, having heard of Tom Foo Yuen through their friends in Redlands, and desiring to take treatment from him. They all received great benefit from their treatment and formed a very high opinion of his character and abilities. They began to invite him to remove to Los Angeles, saying that he was so skillful in the cure of chronic diseases that he was certainly a Godsend to the world, and ought not to hide himself in a small place. They agreed that he ought to remove to a larger city where a greater number of people could profit by his skill. His business associate heard so much of this talk that he gradually become convinced that they ought to make the change desired by the patrons from Los Angeles, and the consequence was that they removed to Los Angeles in June, 1895.

Not long after this removal to Los Angeles, Dr. P. C. Remondino of San Diego, at that time president of the Southern California Medical Association, took occasion to make a bitter attack upon the Chinese System of Medicine in the course of which he made the vulgar charge, which has been disproved hundreds of times, that Chinese physicians are in the habit of using unclean things, toads, lizards and other disgusting materials in their practice. This attack naturally aroused Tom Foo Yuen's resentment, and he replied in an elaborate article published in the Los Angeles Times for August 15, 1895. Dr. Remondino rejoined with another article, to which Tom Foo Yuen also replied, and the argument attracted a great deal of attention. We do not propose to reproduce these articles, as this discussion is now ancient history. But, on this occasion, as before, Foo's American friends rallied to his support, both those who had previously given testimonials in his favor at Redlands, and others. And, in order to show the high esteem in which he was already held by those who knew him best, we reprint herein these testimonials. The reader will notice that they effectually dispose of the principal question raised by Dr. Remondino in his printed articles, and show that only pure, herbal substances have ever been employed by Tom Foo Yuen in his practice. The testimonials are as follows:

J. R. Campbell, for twenty years or more a reputable citizen of San Bernardino county, and at present a resident of Redlands, says: "There is no truth in his (Dr. Remondino's) statement that the educated Chinese physician uses stuffs as vile as Dr. Remondino claims. I have taken directly from his laboratory many packages of Dr. Foo's herbs and cooked them at home. I have closely examined the formulas, and they were composed of nothing but roots, berries, nuts, leaves and twigs, and the results of taking his medicines have been most satisfactory. Dr. Foo is a gentleman of refinement, and can be relied on."

H. B. Ruggles, also of Redlands, says: "I have taken many packages of herbs from Dr. Foo's office, and am emphatic in declaring that nothing in the form of dry herbs could be more clean and pure. Not a sign of any animal product or any similar substance appeared."

A. A. Elge of Bald Butte, Mont., says: "While a patient of Dr. Foo's I frequently viewed the compounding of his medicines, having heard that Chinese used questionable articles, and I satisfied myself that the rumors were unfounded, and that Dr. Foo used nothing but herbs. Their great beauty lies in their wonderful cures."

W. A. Hallowell, Jr., of Ontario, says: "In regard to the address of Dr. Remondino on Chinese medicine, I think it a great exaggeration and devoid of facts. The writer evidently knows nothing of the true system of medicine as practiced by the educated Chinese. I have personally seen in Dr. Foo's laboratory, hundreds of doses of medicine steeped and put up for different persons, and I have never seen any of the vile ingredients used that are mentioned in the address of Dr. Remondino, but they were composed entirely of barks, roots, berries, leaves and herbs, and all in a nice, clean condition."

Miss L. B. Nettleton of Redlands says: "I have taken Dr. Foo's medicines for over a year, and carefully examined each package of medicine, but found nothing but herbs, clean and prepared in a neat manner."

Mrs. J. A. Hendrickson of Redlands, says: "I have been familiar with Dr. Foo's methods for over two years, and have made a hundred doses of tea from the herbs compounded in his laboratory. If anything of such a nature as Dr. Remondino speaks of had been used I surely would have found it out, for I have always had free access to the laboratory. In my opinion, if any one had found such things as eyes, toenails, lizards, snakeskins and other substances too vile to quote, they must have been afflicted with snakes in their boots."

J. W. Symmes, of Redlands, says: "The education of our home doctors seems to be the barrier to their receiving the same benefits of the genuine Chinese physician's skill that the less wise have enjoyed. It is said that an educated man should make such statements in regard to your medicine without first having proven to himself that they were truthful. Nothing of the vegetable kind could be purer than your medicines. I gained my knowledge from nearly a year's experience as a patient of Dr. Foo, and direct observation in his laboratory. The results of his treatment are convincing evidence that Dr. Foo possesses a wonderful fund of scientific knowledge, or else he is the superior of all guessers of the medical profession. The 'taking card' in Dr. Foo's system of treatment is his success."

Levi Carter, of Ceres, Cal., says: "If Dr. Remondino had been as thorough in his investigation of the subject as a man who undertakes to enlighten the public should be, he would have gathered material for an address to the medical association that would have been truly edifying to lovers of the truth and of incalculable value to the afflicted. For, to my mind, there is sufficient evidence in and around Redlands of your skill and the purity of your medicines to convince any sane person that Dr. Foo's superior is not to be found among practitioners of modern methods of medication. The medicines I received from you were purely vegetable, presented a neat appearance, and the effects were wonderfully beneficial. In my opinion Dr. Foo cannot be extolled too highly."

Thomas Stewart says: "I take pleasure in giving my humble opinion of Dr. Foo as a physician. In the first place, his diagnosis of my case, it being by the pulse alone, seemed to me wonderful, he thereby locating my trouble exactly. On my first visit to the doctor I was perfectly helpless, not being able to take a single step without assistance. My legs were swollen to such an extent from the knees to the toes that no joints were visible. This he entirely reduced in five days' treatment, and the swelling has not returned in the least. He explained to me the nature of the different poisons in my system, and how he would expel them, which he did in fourteen days' treatment. What most surprised me was the simplicity of his treatment and the purity of his medicines, they being entirely vegetable—herbs, roots, berries and barks. This I can verify from personal observation. I am now, after a little over four weeks' treatment, as well as ever, except a little weakness in my legs, which are daily improving. My friends who came to see me when I was ill now tell me they never expected to see me out again.

"I regard the success of my treatment as more than wonderful in view of the fact that I am advanced in age. I have received treatment from other doctors, but instead of improving I continued to grow worse until I took treatment from Dr. Foo. One who has suffered the excruciating pains from rheumatism alone can imagine the joy of my experience in being cured.

"I shall certainly advise any friends of mine, who may need a physician, no matter what their disease may be, to consult Dr. Foo of Redlands, Cal.

"Very respectfully yours, THOS. STEWART."

From this time Tom Foo Yuen's business and popularity grew very rapidly. And, as his skill became better known, he attracted to his office a very high class of patronage, intelligent, thinking men and women, who were independent enough to decide for themselves and to believe the evidences of their own senses, in spite of their inherited and acquired prejudices. These ladies and gentlemen saw that, no matter what theorists might say, the actual, undeniable results of the herbal treatment were many remarkable cures. Patrons continued to come from San Bernardino, Redlands and Riverside and the country surrounding those interior cities, and finally became so numerous that Tom Foo Yuen for some time made a trip to San Bernardino every two weeks, in order to see these patrons.

His experience with the American doctor in San Bernardino was very similar to his experience with members of the fraternity in Redlands and Los Angeles. Dr. C. A. Stoddard of San Bernardino apparently became alarmed at Foo's growing success in that city, and caused his arrest on a charge of the illegal practice of medicine. The case was thrown out of court by the justice before whom it was brought, Foo having in the meantime given bonds for appearance; but, as usual, it created a great deal of discussion among physicians and their patients in the newspapers. An open letter to Dr. Stoddard was published in the San Bernardino Times-Index for December 28, 1895. This letter stated concisely Tom Foo Yuen's position in reference to the charges brought against him, and attracted much attention at the time. It is an able defence of the right of every man who is skilled in healing; to use his skill for the benefit of the unfortunate among mankind who are afflicted with disease.

T. Foo Yuen has continued to reside in Los Angeles since his removal to that city from Redlands in 1895. For several years his home, and that of the institution of which he is the head, has been at 903 S. Olive street. In the course of time the Foo and Wing Herb Company was incorporated, as an incorporation seemed to be the best form of association for conducting the constantly growing business.

T. Foo Yuen and his associates have at different times prepared and published many articles dealing with medical topics from the Oriental point of view. A few of these are reprinted in this volume and will doubtless be of interest to the reader. A project upon which Foo has bestowed much thought is the establishment in America of a College of Oriental Medicine, at which the merits of the Chinese system of herbal treatment could be taught to American students. Some further reference will be made to this subject in the succeeding pages.

A College of Oriental Medicine in Los Angeles—A Long Cherished Plan of T. Foo Yuen's—Encouragement From Many of His Patrons.

HIGH PRAISE FROM A MINISTER

ON THE ANCIENT ART OF HEALING THE SICK.

Rev. James Bracewell Pays Tribute to the Wonderfull Skill of the Celebrated Oriental Imperial Physician, Tom Foo Yuen.

He Is the Best Fitted Man to Establish and Preside Over an Oriental Medical College in This Country—Something New in America.

A remarkable thing about the Oriental system of medicine is its growing popularity in the United States. Of course, everybody is prejudiced against anything Chinese, as we forget that there are all classes among this people, as among other races, the rich and the poor, the small and the great, the educated and the ignorant. We of America judge the whole nation by the standard of its lowest class, the laborers who come to our shores and undertake menial employments. We rarely meet the men of education and influence, and know comparatively little about them. The surprise of an American is therefore great when he finds that herbs imported from China and prescribed by a Chinese physician have cured him of some painful and perhaps chronic malady. It has occurred to many people who have had this experience that the American people at large ought to have the benefit of these remedies. It seems like a very plain and simple proposition that if there are medicines not in use among our own physicians which are nevertheless of great value, those medicines ought to be brought to their attention and they ought to be induced to investigate their merits, and, if found satisfactory, to adopt them in their practice. Dr. Foo is willing to assist in this effort, and many of his patrons believe that it would be successful. The intention is to establish a College of Oriental Medicine, at which the principles of this system shall be taught to all who care to study them, just as the methods of other systems of medicine are taught in other schools. Among the many men who, from the favorable opinion which they have formed of this method of healing, are desirous of seeing such a school established in Los Angeles, is the Rev. James Bracewell of Ontario, a gentleman of intelligence and culture who has had opportunity to study the merits of this system, and has been very favorably impressed by them. His letter was originally published in the Los Angeles papers, December 22, 1896, and is as follows.

ONTARIO, Cal., Dec. 8, 1896.

To the Public:

I became acquainted with T. Foo Yuen, the celebrated Chinese physician, about three years ago, and in conversing with him I learned much of his methods of diagnosing diseases and the medicines he uses in his practice. I was much surprised to learn that his only method of locating diseases in the human body, and the strength or virulence of the disease, was by simply feeling the pulse. So to satisfy myself and remove all doubts in regard to the matter, I put the doctor to the test and found that he exactly described my condition. I also talked with several persons present who had been treated by him and had been entirely cured of diseases of long standing, or in a fair way of complete recovery. Those parties all expressed the utmost confidence in his ability as a skillful physician; in fact, so far as I could learn, all those cases were chronic, difficult and unyielding, where the ordinary means as employed by our American doctors had utterly failed to effect a cure.

For the sake of suffering humanity in the United States, where diseases are so prevalent, I should be glad if Dr. Foo should establish a medical college in this country, where the Chinese system of medicine as taught in the Imperial Medical College of Peking, China, could be taught, and thereby a knowledge of the ancient art of healing the sick could be spread abroad in this country. Many people are very much prejudiced against the Chinese system of medicine and the methods employed by Chinese physicians. This is to be accounted for by the fact that most people fail to distinguish between the ignorant and in many cases fraudulent Chinese physicians and those who are educated, intelligent and conscientious. All the graduates of the Imperial Medical College of Peking are very well educated, so I am well informed from the best authority, but there are only thirty of those physicians in the vast Chinese empire, and their practice is confined mostly to their own countrymen.

Dr. Foo is a graduate of the Imperial Medical College of Peking, China. He is a nephew of the distinguished Li Po Tai, formerly of San Francisco, Cal., from whom he received much information as to the difference in the physical make-up between the man of Oriental birth and the man of Occidental birth, the difference being caused by climate, soil, food and environment, and all these things cause different diseases, or modifications of the same disease, and hence rare skill is required on the part of the Chinese physician to so accurately determine the nature of the disease and the proper remedies to give in each particular case.

Dr. Foo is without a peer among Chinese physicians in the United States.

He has a diploma from the Imperial Medical College at Peking, China, and certificates from the Chinese Consul at San Francisco, all of which are genuine. I believe Dr. Foo is the proper man to establish a Chinese medical college in this country, and thus impart to our people a knowledge of the system of medicine as taught and practiced by learned physicians of China.

At one time the homeopathic physicians were not recognized in this country, but now receive the same recognition as is given to the allopathic physicians.

Dr. Foo being a skilled physician, an educated, conscientious gentleman, is entitled to the same consideration and respect. Our government ought not to discriminate against any man on account of race or place of birth, but accord to all equal rights and equal protection, and we should recognize skill, worth and merit wherever we may find them.

I have written this letter in order to say something in behalf of Dr. Foo and his books and writings.

I should be glad if others who are interested in these matters would lend a helping hand, and thus give encouragement and support to what I consider a worthy and meritorious cause. Yours truly,

REV. JAMES BRACEWELL.

THE COLLEGE OF ORIENTAL MEDICINE.

An Opportunity for Americans—They May Now Acquaint Themselves With the Most Ancient System of Healing Extant.

Rev. Mr. Bracewell's letter attracted a great deal of attention among Foo's numerous friends and acquaintances. Letters from others in favor of the plan of establishing a college soon began to come, showing that the idea was popular with those best qualified to judge of its merits. We give a few of these herewith, as they illustrate the standing which this system has attained among its friends.

Not the least of Foo's accomplishments is his acquaintance with the English language. When he came to America he knew not a word of English, but now he speaks it with surprising clearness, and shows wonderful aptness in learning the exact shades of meaning of new words and in acquiring their pronunciation. This faculty of learning a language which all foreigners find difficulty in acquiring is doubtless due in great part to Foo's overmastering ambition to be the first of his race to impart the secrets of Oriental medicine to the western world. This has been a favorite project with him ever since he first came to this coast, and he is now perfecting arrangements to carry the plan into execution. He proposes to establish a school or college of Oriental medicine, in order that American physicians and others may familiarize themselves with diagnosis by the pulse and with the use of the Chinese herbal remedies, as well as with the philosophy of the system.

To the unthinking, this plan may seem foolish and impracticable. There are always people who are willing to condemn, without investigation, anything that is new to them, especially if it comes from a country which is supposed to be inhabited by barbarians. But it is a striking fact, which cannot be ignored, that those who know T. Foo Yuen best are the most ardent supporters of his plan. It is hardly reasonable to suppose that these people are all mistaken in their ideas of the value of this system of medicine. Some of our own physicians even, who have investigated it, have declared that there is merit both in diagnosis by the pulse and in the use of non-poisonous herbal remedies. Just how far these can be used under American habits of life and ways of thinking may be a question, but many shrewd observers will believe that there are fortunes awaiting the people who are the first to study into these matters and adapt this system to the needs of our civilization.

GREAT BENEFITS TO AMERICANS.

The following is from a lady who has had a very remarkable experience with this system. She says:

LOS ANGELES, Cal., Dec. 15, 1896.

In 1895 my little daughter, Clara, was cured by Dr. Foo of a very long and painful disease, which required a great deal of surgical attention and had been unsuccessfully treated by eight white physicians. They had pronounced the case incurable, and had given her up, but Dr. Foo cured her without the use of instruments and without any pain or danger, simply by the use of herbal remedies and some local applications. The full history of this cure was published in the Los Angeles papers in February, 1896, and I think that everybody will still remember it, as it attracted a great deal of attention at the time.

Not long ago I had a great deal of trouble with neuralgia in the head, with fainting spells. Dr. Foo gave me remedies for these difficulties, which I took for four months and a half, with the result that I was completely cured. My son, Will P. Carr, while working in the mines in Arizona, contracted mineral poison, which took the form of eczema. He could not come to Los Angeles for treatment, but I learned that Dr. Foo is able to treat patients at a distance by means of an excellent list of questions which he has prepared. My son answered these questions carefully and wrote a letter every two weeks telling about his condition as fully as possible. Dr. Foo would send two weeks' medicine at a time, and in this way my son was cured in three months. Then I understood that Dr. Foo's skill can be adapted to all cases both at home and at a distance.

Others of my friends have had similar experiences with Dr. Foo, and all have been satisfied with the results. I am convinced by what I have seen that Dr. Foo must have had a very thorough education in Oriental medicine, which fact is further shown by his position as a member of the faculty of the Imperial Medical College at Peking, China.

I have thought for a long time that some influential person ought to take this system up and introduce it to the notice of the American people, for it is certainly worthy of study.

I have been in hopes that somebody who was qualified would make a strong plea for Dr. Foo's skill and attract students to his system of curing. I believe that this would be a great benefit to the

American people and to the world. I now understand that Rev. Mr. Bracewell has given his opinions for this purpose, and I shall certainly try to help him in every way within my power. I am very glad to see this plan started, and I believe that it will succeed

My own knowledge of Oriental medicine is proved by facts which are so clear that it is impossible for me to question them. These facts are also known by a wide circle of my friends and acquaintances. If there were no other cases of cures except those in my own family I should be fully convinced of the merits of this system. I therefore have no hesitancy in recommending his system, and I am sure that if it can be taught in such a way that our own people can understand the use of these herbal remedies and can learn how to prescribe them for various diseases, a great deal of good will result and many people in all parts of the country will be benefited I hope that the proposed college will be a success. MRS. ANNIE HUMPHERY,
217 East Ann street.

ADVANTAGES OVER OTHER METHODS.

George W. Hazard discusses this subject in the following appreciative letter:

LOS ANGELES, Cal., Dec. 14, 1896.

I have seen the letter written by Rev. James Bracewell of Ontario, published in the Los Angeles Express of December 12, in reference to the establishment in this country of a school of Oriental medicine by T. Foo Yuen. Mr. Bracewell is entirely disinterested in this matter, having derived his favorable opinion of Oriental medicine from personal observation. His motive in recommending the founding of such a school is simply that of doing good to the world, and is prompted by his kindness of heart and his philanthropy as a minister of the gospel. I know Mr. Bracewell and have a high opinion of his character and attainments, which command the respect of all who know him.

His ideas are in accord with those of many others who have personally studied the merits of the Oriental system of medicine and have watched the results of that system, either in their own cases or in the cases of friends and acquaintances. I am aware that it is the fashion, in some quarters, to discredit this system because it comes from a people who are supposed to be inferior in intelligence to the Caucasian race. While I am not inclined to discuss this question at length, yet there are a few well-established facts which indicate that this widely-prevalent opinion is erroneous, and show that this ancient system of medicine is, in many respects, both of theory and of practice, superior to that which is practiced among us at the present time. To discredit it and despise it simply because it has come down to the human race through hundreds of years and because it is practiced by a people who are aliens to us, seems to me a mark not of intelligence, but of foolish national pride, or race prejudice, which prevents us from seeing the good that may exist among other nations.

Take the Chinese ideas of anatomy, for instance, which were originally founded upon the practice of vivisection. These ideas differ in many important particulars from the ideas taught in our own schools. Yet they are so thoroughly rooted in common sense that they appeal at once to the intelligence of all who take the trouble to investigate them without prejudice. The teachings of the Oriental system in reference to the functions of the spleen are an example of this. Physicians of our own race admit that they know nothing about the functions of this organ. They so state in their text-books, and so they inform their medical students. In a controversy over the merits of Chinese medicine about a year and a half ago a prominent physician of Southern California accused T. Foo Yuen of false pretenses because he claimed to know something about the functions of this organ, and ridiculed this claim, saying, in effect, that if this were true Dr. Foo knew more than all the great doctors who have ever lived among civilized races.

I was told recently by a gentleman of intelligence and personal integrity of a case in Southern California in which ignorance of the functions of this organ was a factor in determining the life or death of a patient, Alexander Gordon, the victim of a gunshot wound, accidentally received in the stomach. During an operation the attending physicians came upon the patient's spleen, in the course of their cutting. "We don't know what this is for," they said, "and it isn't of any use to the man, anyhow." So they cut it out and threw it away. The patient died in a few hours. This incident, incredible as it seems to be, was told to me for truth, and, whether it is true or not, it shows the general ignorance of the medical profession as regards the functions of this organ is well understood among all classes.

Now, as God made the human body as it is, He evidently intended the spleen to perform some important function. If it had nothing to do it would not be a part of the human body. It is certainly astounding that students of the human body should remain in ignorance of the functions of this or any other organ, or, being ignorant, should be willing to admit that ignorance, and should deride others for claiming in good faith, to possess knowledge upon this subject.

The Chinese system of anatomy and medicine explains this matter and many others upon which our ideas seem to be indefinite and confused. Dr. Foo has briefly explained the functions of the spleen in chapters from his forthcoming books, already published, and will discuss them more in detail at a later date. The American people are the wonder and admiration of all other nations of the world for their advance and progress in everything outside of the care of their bodies and lives. In matters of trade, finance, transportation, mining, agriculture and everything in which human ingenuity may be applied to mechanical or industrial pursuits, we lead the world. But we, as a nation, are making no advances or improvements upon our own methods of taking care of our health and curing our diseases. This neglected field seems to me the most important field of all, and I think that when a new system of medicine—or at least one which is new to us—is offered to us, we should give it a careful consideration I believe that the profession of medicine is more important today than any other profession, and is less satisfactory as compared with the advances in other professions.

It is not only in theory that the Chinese system of medicine has shown its merits and proved its successes. In results it is equally satisfactory. It is impossible to explain away this fact, which is proved by the testimony of many living witnesses. There is something in the remedies used or the diagnoses which cure where other methods fail. I do not make the absurd claim that this system always cures, or the equally absurd claim that no other system has any good in it, or that all our physicians are ignorant or incompetent, but I do say that in many respects, and in the treatment of many diseases, the Chinese system has advantages over others, as is shown by the results of treatment with the Chinese herbal remedies.

For this reason I am in favor of the establishment of an Oriental college of medicine in Los Angeles, as suggested by Rev. Mr. Bracewell's letter. I believe that a consistent, thorough and unbiased study of the principles underlying this system of medicine would benefit humanity by adding to the sum of human knowledge upon questions of health, which are questions of the very highest importance.

GEORGE W. HAZARD.

LOS ANGELES, Cal., Jan. 4, 1902.

To the Foo & Wing Herb Co.:

Gentlemen:—I desire to inform the public, and especially sufferers from disease, of the remarkable cure you effected in my case. My principal trouble was muscular and inflamatory rheumatism, which came on me while ranching in Colorado six years ago. Since

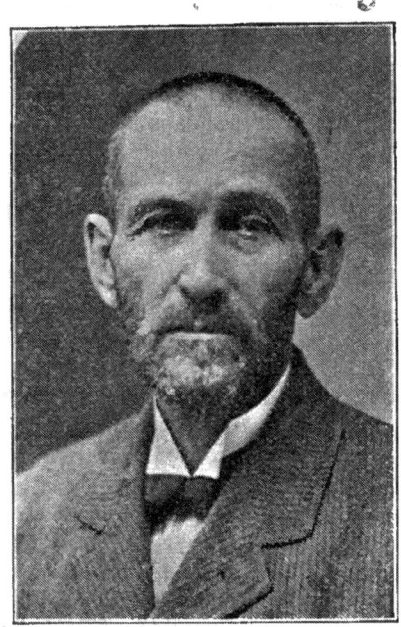

G. W. MOODY.

that time I have suffered much pain and endured many inconveniences from this terrible disease. I sought relief from many eminent doctors—so called—in different parts of the country, but they did me no good. I also visited hot springs at different times, and found no relief from that source, but gradually grew worse, and finally decided to come to Los Angeles, thinking the change in climate might be beneficial, as I had almost despaired of getting relief from any source, and at the end of two months' residence here I was feeling much worse than when I arrived. Fortunately for me, however, about that time I noticed your advertisement in the papers, and, prompted by curiosity, I concluded to call and have an examination, which I did, and after undergoing the wonderful pulse diagnosis by Dr. T. Foo Yuen, I was so surprised, as well as elated over the correctness of the diagnosis, as he described my feelings better than I could have done, that I decided at once to try your herb remedies, as I was convinced after giving me such a correct diagnosis that you were skilled and clever enough to cure my disease; and I am happy to say that I was not disappointed. After taking two and one-half courses of your wonderful herb remedies I find myself relieved from one of the worst diseases that afflicts mankind And I feel better in every way than I have at any time during the past ten years, and feel that I have a new lease of life. When I first came to you I was scarcely able to walk. Now I take long walks daily, and also ride the bicycle and enjoy the exercise. I can cheerfully and conscientiously recommend the Chinese herbal remedies when administered by such skillful and scintific doctors as the members of the Foo and Wing Herb Co.

Yours truly, G W. MOODY,
221 S. Bunker Hill avenue.

A GENERAL LETTER FROM SEVERAL PATRONS SHOWING THAT RESULTS HAVE GIVEN THEM CONFIDENCE.

LOS ANGELES, California.
T. Foo Yuen, City:

Dear Sir: The results of our treatment by the Oriental system of medicine as practiced by you have been very satisfactory to us, and have proved to us that there is great benefit to be derived from the herbal remedies when their use is directed by the care and skill of which you are possessed.

We have also watched the effects of this treatment in other cases of which we have known or which we have seen while we have been your patrons. The favorable results in these cases have inspired confidence in the system and in your skill and ability. These remedies seem to be adapted to a great many different diseases and to be successful in an unusually large proportion of the cases which commence treatment.

We believe that a wider knowledge of the principles of this system would result in great good to invalids and to the world in general. We think that such knowledge ought to be encouraged in every way, and that people ought to be urged to study this system, both in its theories and in the many cases which show its results. We believe that you are well qualified by your skill in the use of these remedies, by your knowledge of the English language, and by your acquaintance with the condition of the treatment of white people, both to teach the theories of the system of medicine and to practice those theories in particular cases, as applied to the treatment of different diseases.

For this reason we are willing to sign this general letter of recommendation as an encouragement to others to study this system, and, if out of health, to test it for themselves. Very truly yours,

MR. H. D. EVEREST, P. O. box 283, Los Angeles.
MR. E. W. SANDISON, 38th and Budlong avenue, Los Angeles.
MRS. T. D. MERRYMAN, 3020 Hoover street, Los Angeles.
COL. E. D. G. MORGAN, Duarte, Cal.
MRS. M. RAYMOND, 1037 S. Broadway, Los Angeles.
MR. A. J. SANBORN, 419 E. Fourth street, Los Angeles.
MR. E. M. WADE, 115½ N. Main street, Los Angeles.
N. VAN ZANDT, Ft. Dodge, Iowa.
MRS. B. HOWARD, 467 C street, San Bernardino, Cal.
MR. J. W. SYMMES, Redlands, Cal.
MR. HENRY F. DE SOUZA, San Jacinto, Cal.
MR. B. J. INWALL, San Jacinto, Cal.
MRS. E. P. HILLMAN, 919 South Broadway.
H. I. ROPER, Station A, Los Angeles.
MRS. S. E. BRYSON, Belmont avenue and Temple street.
A. WILSON, 261 E. Tenth street, Riverside, Cal.
GEO. W. HAZARD, 933 South Broadway.
MRS. A. T. CHUBB, 949 South Broadway.
WM. COGSWELL, 1138 South Flower street.
MISS SADIE M'PHERSON, McPherson, Orange county, Cal.
C. B. GRANNIS, 1508 South Main street.
J. J. TYLER, South Pasadena, Cal.
MRS. P. N. PORTMAN, 501 Temple street, Los Angeles.
F. E. STURGIS, 301 South Broadway, Los Angeles.

C. R. WHEELER, 117 San Pedro street, Los Angeles.
MRS. J. C. RHOADES, Los Angeles.
A. A. DEXTER, JR., Fourth and A streets, San Bernardino, Cal.
MR. and MRS. MAGGA MOTHERSPAW, Del Rosa, Cal.
E. R. VAN DEURSEN, 482 Third street, San Bernardino, Cal.
W. M. WRIGHT, Ontario, Cal.
J. T. BURROWS, San Bernardino, Cal.
E. P. LANE, San Bernardino, Cal.
HENRY B. RUGGLES, Redlands, Cal.
JOHN SCEALEY, Redlands, Cal.
A. J. HENDRICKSON, Redlands, Cal.
J. R. CAMPBELL, Redlands, Cal.
MRS. MATTIE REEDER, Redlands, Cal.
E. C. WARREN, Redlands, Cal.
MRS. FANNIE VAN LEUVEN, 1844 Naud street, Los Angeles, Cal.
MISS B. M. COX, Riverside, Cal.
MRS. C. ELLIS, 623 Tehama street, Los Angeles.
J. B. COURTNEY, 730 Commercial street, Los Angeles.
MRS. J. A. JONES, 1002 Alpine street, Los Angeles.
P. J. BRANNEN, 1301 West Washington street, Los Angeles.
MRS. T. G. KELTY, San Bernardino, Cal.

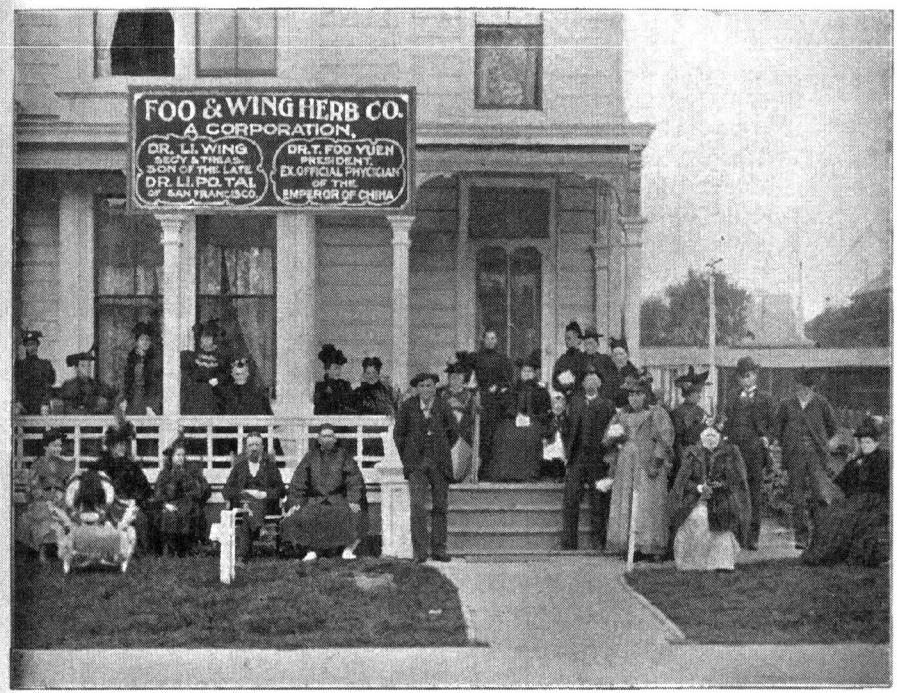

THE FIRST HOME OF THE FOO & WING HERB COMPANY.

The above cut represents the former office of the Foo & Wing Herb Company, together with a few of the many patients who have been benefited by the genuine Oriental System of Medicine. This office was on Broadway, Los Angeles, but, after remaining here for a few months, the company was compelled, by increasing business, to seek larger quarters.

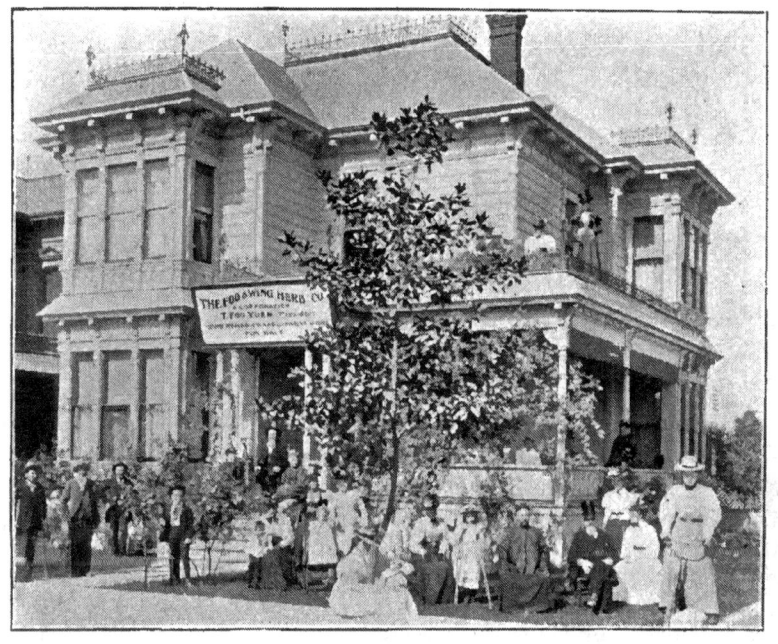

The above cut represents the office and home of the Foo & Wing Herb Company at the present writing, January, 1902. This handsome and commodious building is at No. 903 S. Olive street, one of the finest of the residence streets of Los Angeles. It is convenient to the business center and easily reached by several lines of electric cars. This has been the headquarters of this company for several years past. Should any change in location be made hereafter the fact will be noted in the advertisements of the company in the daily papers of Los Angeles.

CHAPTER V.

TOM LEONG.

Vice-President of the Foo and Wing Herb Company—A Brief Sketch of His Life and Education.

Tom Leong, vice-president of the Foo and Wing Herb Company, is a brother of Tom Foo Yuen, and is, therefore, like him, a descendant of a race of physicians. Tom Leong was born in 1868. Since he came to Los Angeles, a few years ago, he has been an assistant to his brother, who considers his skill in the cure of disease equal to his own. This has been shown by the cure of many difficult cases. For six generations past their family has been a race of physicians, and the remedies which they employ are secrets that have been transmitted from one generation to another and improved as a result of very wide experience. Most of the ancestors of these two men have been physicians of national reputation in their own country.

During his residence in the United States Foo has studied closely the application of his remedies for the cure of Americans, and his brother, Tom Leong, has reaped the benefit of the experience thus acquired. Tom Leong's education, in his own country, was far above that of the ordinary Chinese physician. From the beginning of his education he was an enthusiastic student in all the disorders of the human system. His grandfather was physician to the Emperor of China, and was a man of high rank in his country. His father was the late Dr. T. Gee Son. They taught Tom Leong from the text-books of their profession, which he studied with a degree of intelligence and power of learning far greater than the average. He readily grasped subjects which were very deep and difficult of understanding.

Tom Leong commenced his studies at school at the age of six years, and continued these for thirteen years, when he was graduated from the common schools. Three years later he was graduated from the high school. He then commenced in earnest the study of medicine at a hospital conducted in Canton by his father, who had returned to Canton after living in San Francisco for several years as an associate physician with Li Po Tai, during which time he cured many white people. This building was surrounded by a park. In the front of the building was the office where the patients were received.

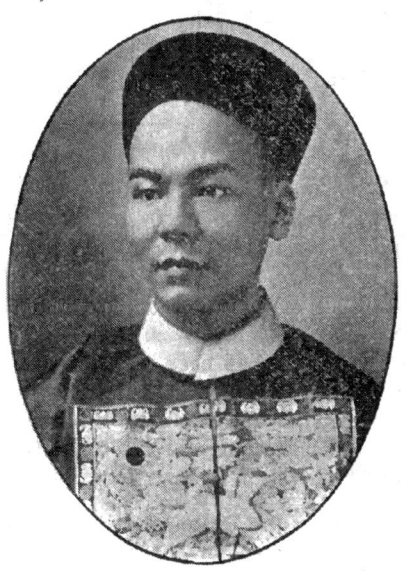

There was also a library filled with the books comprised in the course of medical instruction, and in this room Tom Leong spent most of his time, every day for three years in very earnest study. During this time he was not allowed to go away to visit his friends or to go home or to engage in anything that would distract his mind from his work. His mother alone was permitted to see him, but she had to come to him as he was not permitted to go to see her. His only vacation during the whole year was a period of about ten days during the New Year, when he was permitted to go home and see his relatives and friends. Every Sunday was a day of rest but, although Tom Leong could rest from his work, yet he could not go out, except into the park, where he took his daily exercise. Yet, although he was very industrious, the confinement and close application to study did not injure his health.

Tom Leong followed this course of instruction for three years to the great satisfaction of his teachers. And, after he had attained proficiency in the lessons taught in the books, they commenced to teach him diagnosis by the pulse. He was now granted more freedom, was permitted to go into the office where the patients were accustomed to assemble for examination and to go to see his friends. His teachers were not so severe as during the first three years. But he still studied the medical books very carefully and also learned the use of the different remedies. In the course of six years he had studied the ancient medical books, written four thousand years ago, and also all the important works on medicine written since that time. He then became versed in the special remedies which had been handed down in his family from generation to generation. The next step was to commence to prepare prescriptions, when his father was busy, and in this way he entered upon the active practice of medicine.

Tom Leong's father was anxious to have his son very skillful in medicine, more so, even, than himself. He therefore sent him to study with a physician named Fay Pak Hong, who was the most prominent physician in all China. He lived in the city of Mangho, near Shanghai, in the province of Gong Nam, district of Sou Chou. After this celebrated physician had seen Tom Leong and had given him an examination, he declared that he was already so proficient that he himself could teach him only a little, and that the remedies which he understood were better even than those which had been handed down in his own family. So Fay Pak Hong made him a teacher over three boys of his own in order that they might get the benefit of an understanding of the remedies which had been handed down from father to son in Tom Leong's family. In return, he taught Tom Leong the secrets of his own remedies, thus improving both systems.

Tom Leong remained with Fay Pak Hong for two years and then entered the Imperial Medical College at Peking, where he studied for three years and was then graduated, thus becoming an Imperial doctor. He then returned to Canton. At that time the Foo and Wing Herb Company had just been incorporated, and the members of this company wanted Tom Leong to undertake the general supervision of the preparation of their remedies in China, because they could be manufactured of a better quality in China than in San Francisco, as the choicest herbs could be obtained there more easily. The remedies prepared by Tom Leong have been found very efficient and have made the work of the Foo and Wing Company more successful than before.

The Foo and Wing Herb Company was incorporated in 1897, and after acting as its agent in Canton for two years, during which time the company was very prosperous, Tom Leong then came to Los Angeles as an assistant to T. Foo Yuen, the president of the company.

We print testimonials of a few of the cures that have been made by Tom Leong in Los Angeles, also some articles on a few phases of Oriental medicine prepared by Tom Leong and his brother, T. Foo Yuen, working together. Under the direction of his brother also, Tom Leong has made a study of the special uses of the remedies in the treatment of the diseases of white people, and adapting them to the white man's ways of life. Tom Leong's diploma from the Imperial Medical College at Peking is substantially the same as T. Foo Yuen's, and for that reason we do not reproduce it in these pages. But we have given his certificate from the Chinese Consul-General at San Francisco both in Chinese and in English, in order that all may understand it.

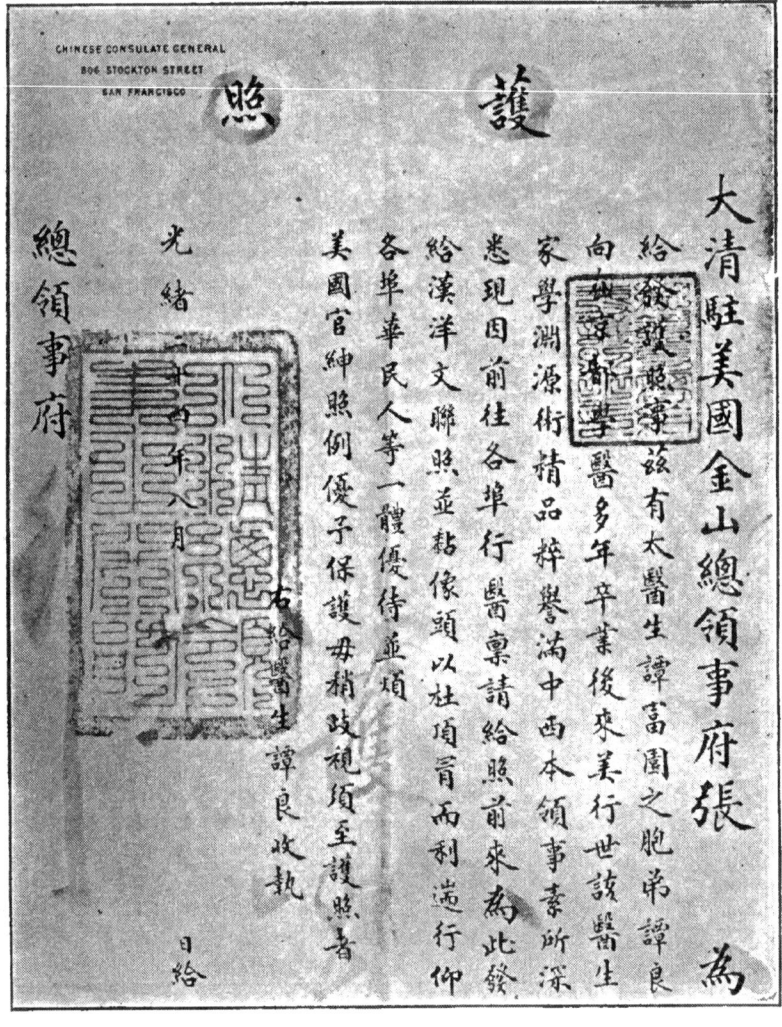

FAC-SIMILE OF TOM LEONG'S CERTIFICATE FROM THE CHINESE CONSUL-GENERAL.

San Francisco California
September 19th 1898

This is to certify that I Chang Yin Tung, His Imperial Majesty's Consul General to the port of San Francisco am personally acquainted with Dr. Tom Leong whose photograph is hereto attached.

I know Dr. Tom Leong to have been a member of the Imperial College of Medicines in Peking and to be a graduate thereof.

He has been practicing his profession in this city for several years and achieved great success.

He is the younger brother of Dr. T. Foo Yuen.

Chang Yin Tung
H. I. C. M's Consul General

TRANSLATION OF TOM LEONG'S CERTIFICATE FROM THE CHINESE CONSUL-GENERAL.

CHAPTER VI.

SOME TOPICS FROM ORIENTAL MEDICINE.

Lessons on Anatomy and on the Cause and Origin of Diseases—The Medical Profession in China—The Herbal Remedies—Vivisection Among the Chinese.

These articles were first published in the Los Angeles papers. They are certainly very unique, and are the result of patient investigation by the learned men of one of the most observing peoples on the face of the earth. The more these lessons are studied, the more fully the force of their reasoning is impressed upon the mind of the student.

LESSON NO. 1—THE CHINESE SYSTEM OF ANATOMY.

In the Chinese medical books are described all the remedies which benefit the human system in such a way that everybody may understand. The question then arises: How do the remedies benefit the system? This is a matter that has puzzled very many people of all countries. Even the common doctors of China, those who are not very well educated, cannot understand the reason of this. I will explain why this is so. The excellent reason is given in books written four thousand years ago. The grammar of these books is very hard, and the reasoning is so deep that the common doctor cannot learn. He studies modern and very easy books, but he cannot comprehend philosophy. Many hundred years ago a few very well educated doctors understood everything, but they never had their profound reasoning translated into easy language, and they never had their many hundred books condensed by searching out and separating the essential parts and showing them to all the world.

English people who have lived a good many years in China, and have tried to translate the Chinese medical books, have found them very hard to learn and translate. They have gone part way and stopped when half done, and have found no one suitable to explain these books to them. And because they have not found men sufficiently well educated to explain these books, they have not been able to simplify them. This is because the Chinese language is more difficult to learn than any other in the whole world, and because the medical works which were written four thousand years ago are more difficult than any other books in the Chinese language.

A NEW LESSON ON ANATOMY.

Speaking of anatomy, I suppose that the subject has long been written in the books of all civilized nations. Therefore I need not speak about it here in detail, but I will say a few words here regarding the Chinese system of anatomy. In my chapter or lesson on this subject some parts of the reasoning are like anatomy, some parts are different from anatomy. I cannot always find the proper name in English, but can say Chinese anatomy.

THE FUNCTIONS OF THE FIVE VITAL ORGANS.

I cannot write all of this lesson here because it is too long, but the five kinds of vital organs belong to the five kinds of elements. I shall try to explain the lungs first. The lungs belong to the mineral element. They are in the upper part of the chest. They look like an umbrella. They are connected with the nostrils. They have eight leaves or lobes, six in front and two in the back. There are nine divisions of the pipe through the throat which connect the lungs with the nose and are called in English the trachea. The lungs are joined to the heart by large veins. The power in the outside heat of the lungs can control the air of the body and the power in the inside heat can control the large intestine, and the large intestine belongs to the mineral element.

THE HEART.

Next I shall speak of the heart. This organ belongs to the fire element. It lies just above the diaphragm. There is a close connection between the heart and the tongue, so that when the heart wishes to speak the tongue will follow. The natural heat or influence of the heart can control the eye, the nose, the ear and the tongue alike and altogether. And the seven affections have their seat in the heart. When the man wakes up the power from the heart is furnished to the brain; when the man sleeps the brain power returns to the heart. The power which is within the heart controls the small intestines which also belong to the fire element. The power of the heart through the outside controls the actions of the body by the arteries which carry the blood from the heart through the body. The blood is then of a red color, and it returns to the heart through the veins and is dark. The heart case protects the heart and belongs to the fire element, too, and the power of the heart case goes through the natural heat between the two kidneys, where is the seat of life. Some books say that life is in the brain; some books say that it is in the heart; but the heart and the brain and the kidneys are all connected by the current of air through the natural heat, and all make up one family.

THE SPLEEN.

Now let us speak of the spleen, which belongs to the earth element. This organ lies on the outside of the stomach, under the heart, and its place is near the left side, but the air power goes through the right side, because we can feel the spleen pulse in the right hand. The spleen catches the impulse from the food and liquid taken into the stomach, which we call the food and liquid air, and sets up an action like the balance-wheel of a watch. The heat from the spleen can draw the liquid from the gall, which goes through the food and liquid in the stomach and causes it to be digested. The spleen is connected with the mouth. The power of the spleen on the inside controls the stomach, and the stomach belongs to the earth element. The power goes through the outside and controls the flesh of the body.

THE LIVER.

Next we will speak of the liver. This belongs to the vegetable element, and has seven lobes. It lies in the right side near the stomach, but the power and the air and the pulse go through the left side, because the liver pulse is found in the left hand.

The liver is closely connected with the eye. The power on the inside controls the gall, which belongs to the vegetable element. The power of the liver on the outside controls the nerves of the body.

THE KIDNEYS.

I will try to speak of the kidneys. These belong to the water element and are closely connected with the ear. There are two kidneys, which lie at the base of the spine, one on each side. The pulse follows the spine to the brain, and the kidneys furnish juices to the brain. This is shown because the natural juices of the kidneys are white, the marrow of the spine is white, and the natural juices of the brain are white. And all of these three, the kidneys, the spine and the brain, make one family. The power from the brain inside controls the bladder, which belongs to the water element, and the power on the outside controls the bones of the body and goes between the two kidneys (through the natural heat), and the resulting power belongs to the fire element. And that heat can warm the lower, middle and upper parts of the vital organs.

DIGESTION AND NUTRITION.

I shall try to explain the stomach and the conditions of digestion. When food and liquid are taken into the stomach, then the spleen lies on the outside of the stomach and sets up an action like the balance-wheel of a watch, and causes the digestive processes by agitating the air in the stomach and spleen and by extracting a fluid, from which the blood and all other natural juices of the body are produced. This fluid is of a dark color as taken by the spleen, and is sent by the force of the spleen to the lungs, where it is purified. And then it passes through the lower part, drop by drop, like the falling of rain in a shower. It is distributed to all portions of the body. The power thus derived from the lungs produces all the growth of the skin; that from the heart causes all the action of the body, through the blood; the power of the spleen produces all of the flesh of the body and furnishes all the strength of the body; the liver produces all of the nerves, and the kidneys produce all of the bones. There are five prime vital organs, but these explanations are not full and complete in reference to the growth and control of the body in its different parts.

I will give you an example or illustration of this growth and control. The human body is like unto the earth and the sky. You see how, after a rainstorm, the sun causes the evaporation of the moisture in the earth, which causes clouds, and rushes to the sky, making fog and rain, which falls to the earth producing vegetation. The sun also draws the dampness up again, which makes more clouds, which rush again to the sky, and the clouds make more rainfall, which falls down to the earth, again producing vegetation, giving and taking indefinitely. The spleen is like unto the earth; the lungs are like unto the sky, and the power keeps going from one to the other.

THE QUESTION OF SLEEP.

An interesting question is: "What makes a person sleep?" I will explain this. The starting point in the circulation of the human body is at and from the kidneys to the heart and from the heart to the kidneys. There is a current to and from the kidneys to the heart and from the heart to the kidneys an interchange of air or power, between these two organs, which is perpetual in life. If the current of air between these organs is broken, death ensues instantly. Also there is another kind of air to the kidneys and heart, which manifests its power over the system when the man lies down to sleep. The mind becomes quiet, and then the brain power returns to the heart. Then the second power of the heart expands and rushes to the kidneys, and the second power, or current, of the kidneys expands and rushes to the heart. Then the man sleeps, and if the current of air continues strong there will be good rest.

When there is excessive brain labor this affects the power, which is not strong, and when the current of air makes weak connection, the sleep is very poor. The brain, the heart and the kidneys make one family.

Every one who studies the functions of the vital organs should understand that they perform their functions by the natural power of air. This power can control the blood; the blood cannot control the air. You can see this from the bladder, which makes a little hole into the lower part, but none in the upper part, for the fluids to enter. And the small intestines perform their functions naturally in the same way. The refuse goes through the large intestines and the water goes through the bladder by air power. Any one can get the bladder of a cow or hog for examination. You may turn the lower hole up, and although the water may be full inside not one drop will run down. It all keeps inside. But the power of air can make the water go into the bladder, although there is not a visible place for it to enter. Sometimes the small intestine fails to perform its natural function and does not carry off the water and fluids. Then the water goes through the large intestine and causes sickness.

LESSON NUMBER TWO.

The Cause and Origin of Diseases—Three Prime Sources—Their Influence Upon the Human System Traced and Explained.

There are three prime sources from which the diseases common to mankind originate. The first of these includes such influences as are without and independent of the body. There are six forms of air, namely: Wind, cold, sun heat, damp air, dry air and fire air. The second sources comprises those influences which cause ill health from within the make-up of the individual. There are seven of these, namely: Joy, anger, overwork, study, grief, fright and fear. These are the excessive seven affections. The third source of disease includes those influences which are neither entirely within nor without the make-up of the individual. They include improper food and liquids, fire, hot or cold water and the bites of insects and animals.

Of the six forms of injurious air, the first, wind from the sky, is slow in its effects upon the system. There are a good many different kinds of this air. The second form, cold air, is from the earth. This may cause sickness quickly. There are also a good many kinds of this air. Both of these forms are indispensable to man, yet both are sometimes very destructive and cause the worst forms of disease of any from this source. The ancient medical works tell of 193 kinds of sickness from wind and cold. They work together, but cause atmospheric conditions known by many different names. The third form is sun-heat, which causes many diseases, among which is sunstroke. The fourth form is damp air, and is that which is found in low altitudes and about swamps, and soon after rainstorms. This is the external source and origin of malaria. The fifth form, dry air, is caused by atmospheric changes. This will produce dryness in the throat and mouth, redness of the eyes, and inflammation in other parts of the body. The sixth form, fire air, is a poisonous condition of the atmosphere, and the worst form of this air causes cholera; but other forms cause lighter epidemics. This form of injurious air causes death very quickly, while all the others work destruction slowly.

EFFECTS OF THE EMOTIONS.

An excess of any mental emotion causes disease. Anger affects the heart and liver. Petulance shortens life. Overwork injures the nerves and the bones, and produces an impaired circulation of the blood. Excessive study seriously injures the heart and spleen. Grief also weakens the heart. Fear affects the gall and prevents the secretion of sufficient gall liquid. It also weakens the heart. Fear cannot be driven away. Sudden and intense fright will rupture the gall sack and confuse the seven affections, completely unbalancing the mind and causing insanity,

Among the third causes of disease are eating and drinking improper foods and liquids. Roasted or fried meats cause inflammation and a desire to drink often. Eating more meats than vegetables causes indigestion. Drinking cold drinks and eating raw fruits cause damp air in the system. The inflammation and damp air will lock hands and cause malaria and severe illness. This form of malaria produced internally, is unlike that produced in the open air and inhaled. But it invites an external form, and the two together cause severe forms of disease.

Diseases may commence in the liver and involve the stomach; or they may commence in the stomach and involve the lungs, or they may commence in the kidneys and involve the liver. They may commence in any of the internal organs and involve the skin, the external surface of the body. Disease that commences in the skin, flesh, nerves, cords or muscles will sooner or later involve the internal organs.

The symptoms of disease may be the same in two or more people, yet the causes be entirely different. And a single cause may manifest itself in a number of ways; thus, either headache, backache, stomachache, boneache, toothache or distress of the lungs may be due to the same cause.

Although all men look very much alike and have the same members and organs, yet no two are exactly alike or possess the same degree of external power, which is strength, or of internal power, which is vitality.

The five vital organs are the heart, liver, spleen, lungs and kidneys. The heart-case, gall, stomach, large intestines, small intestines and bladder are agents for the vital organs. The seven affections—joy, anger, grief, pleasure, laughter, hatred and desire—control the vital organs, but have no influence over the six agents of the five vital organs. When either of the five vital organs is the seat of disease the difficulty is more serious than it would be if seated in either of the six sub-organs.

All internal organs have muscles and pulse connecting with the extremities of the body.

FOUR METHODS OF HEALING.

There are four principal methods of healing: First, by warming the blood; second, by cleansing the system; third, by strengthening, and fourth, by purging.

The Chinese system of medicine is taught in branches, such as diseases of children, diseases of women, diseases of men, and diseases of the bones, including injuries to them. Each of these branches requires from three to four years to learn. To acquire a thorough knowledge of medicine and to be able to pass an examination at the Imperial College of Medicine at Peking requires fourteen years of the most arduous labor that ever students of any profession in any country are subjected to. Even then the recipient of a diploma from the college often fails to receive the signature of the Emperor to his diploma because he fails to pass a second and very severe examination before His Majesty.

MEDICAL HISTORY IN CHINA.

A BRIEF HISTORY OF ITS ORIGIN AND PROGRESS---A CALLING HELD IN ESPECIAL HONOR AMONG THE CHINESE.

EARLY PHYSICIANS WHO BECAME EMPERORS---THE FOUNDERS OF THE GREAT IMPERIAL COLLEGE AT PEKIN.

Mrs. Alice Rollins Crane, a well-known writer and journalist, formerly of Los Angeles, now a resident of Dawson City, in the Klondike, once had an interesting interview with T. Foo Yuen, in reference to the Imperial Medical College at Peking. Mrs. Crane stated that she had recently heard a Chinamen say that there is no Imperial Medical College in China. This remark brought out the following discussion of the subject. T. Foo Yuen laughed at the statement and said:

"Did that man say that? He doesn't know the history of the Chinese medical books. The people of some other country might, perhaps say that there is no Imperial Medical College in China, because they do not know the conditions and customs in regard to the medical colleges of the Chinese. But there is no excuse for a Chinaman saying this. Again, some one might have said this twenty years ago, but there is no reason for saying it now when people ought to know better.

"The truth is that the Imperial Medical College was founded four thousand years ago. This college is in Peking, and is within the walls of the great inclosure known as 'The Emperor's World.'

This college is near the front door of the Emperor's palace. This front door is called in the Chinese language Di Ching Mung. The college is on Tong Bew Boy street. On the right of the Imperial Medical College is the office of an official whom we may call an 'almanac officer.' He has charge of all the computations and predictions in regard to the weather, the movements of the heavenly bodies, etc., etc., and corresponds to the American weather bureau. The college is on the right of this building and is next to the corner of the wall surrounding the inclosure. Soldiers always stand before the front door of the college to keep the common people from going in. Only high officials, such as judges, are permitted to enter, because the common people do not understand the regulations which govern the college.

"While I was a student at the Imperial Medical College and before I graduated, many judges and high officials came to take my treatment. Among those who took my treatment and with whom I became well acquainted was Judge Li Yung Yew, who came to San Francisco to be consul-general there, and gave me a certificate of my standing at the Imperial Medical College. This judge says that the Chinese call this college Ti Yee Yun, but that the English name, as nearly as can be translated, is Imperial Medical College, although the customs and ways of teaching in this college are a little different from the English method.

"And now to speak of the commencement of the medical college, four thousand years ago. The first doctor was a holy man named Son Non. He commenced the use of herbal remedies, and there was much benefit to the world from these, that all the people voted to make him Emperor. The second doctor was named Wong Ti. He commenced to explain anatomy and the use of medicines, and he wrote two different kinds of books. The title of the first book was Ling Su Kin, and the title of the other was Su Man Kin. These books continued the work which Sun Tong had commenced, and brought so much benefit into the world, that everybody voted for Wong Day to be Emperor in his turn. And while he was Emperor he built up the Imperial Medical College. And the name of the first president was Kee Ba, who had a large faculty with him as associate physicians and teachers. One of these was Su Su, another Su Yu, and another was Louen Kong, and another was Chung Man. These four put more power into the two books which Wong Day had written and completed them. So it was required all through China that every

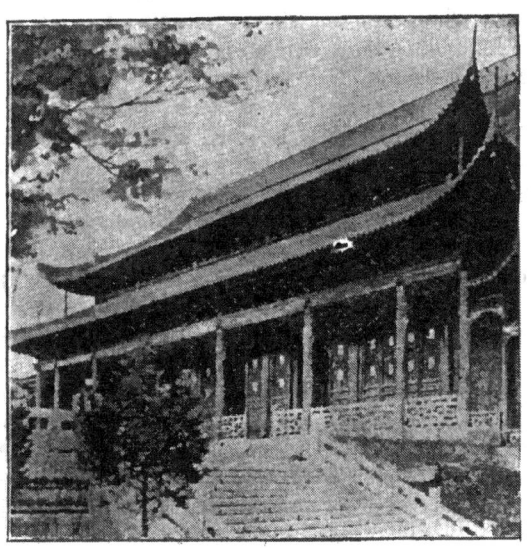

PORTION OF IMPERIAL MEDICAL COLLEGE
AT PEKIN, CHINA.

doctor must be learned in these books and the teachings of them is very skillful indeed. But the grammar and construction of the language is very deep and difficult. This is true of any Chinese book, but the grammar of these medical books is harder than that of any other book in China.

ANCIENT LAWS REGULATING THE PROFESSION.

"So for many years the doctors were compelled to pass examinations in these books and all the very well educated doctors were sought out and divided into two classes, and they were called doctors of the first or second class. They were all called official, or judge, doctors. All of the doctors in the first class were kept in the Imperial Medical College for three years to learn more. They, therefore, stood much higher than the others, and were called physicians to the Emperor. The second-class doctors were permitted to go home, and were called doctors to take care of the people. And for all this time there was a law to regulate the practice of medicine, just as there is among English-speaking people. If a man could not pass the examination, he could not call himself a doctor. But after the time of the tenth Emperor they found this law too severe, and they permitted students to graduate by quick and easy examinations, because the Chinese people had grown so fast that they could not furnish enough doctors to take care of the common people. So they suspended the operation of the law and permitted anybody to be called doctor. But only the graduates from the Imperial Medical College were permitted to be physicians to the Emperor, and these must have passed the examination the same as before. From that time until now, there has been no closing of the doors of the Imperial Medical College. It has always been in operation. Whenever there has been a change of Emperors there has been some change in other laws and customs, but they never changed the management of the Imperial Medical College, which is still conducted in the same way as the first.

THE MORE MODERN WAY.

"But since the law regulating the profession of medicine was changed almost all the students have chosen to learn from easy books, and all have wanted to learn quickly and the things that were handiest. So that there have not been many people to learn from the books written four thousand years ago, which are so hard. This matter is getting worse all the time, and the doctors are becoming of a cheaper class. The English people, who have been building up Hongkong, employ doctors on the steamship lines and in the hospitals. Formerly they tried to have one English and one Chinese doctor in each place, and for this purpose they gave examinations for the Chinese doctors for a long time, but they could not find any Chinese doctors who could explain anatomy and the causes of diseases. This was because the educated Chinese doctors would not go to take these examinations held by the English, for the reason that the systems and knowledge were different, and also the medicines employed. From that time, the English people in China have detested the Chinese doctors because they have seen and known only the poorest and cheapest of them, and those that have no education; and after a time, on the steamers and in the hospitals conducted by the English, only English doctors were employed, and they stopped employing Chinese doctors.

LACK OF GOOD PHYSICIANS IN CHINA.

"For these reasons, anywhere through China, in the course of a few hundred miles, perhaps one, two or three very good native doctors will be found, and these perform so many wonderful cures, that the English people are surprised. They look on in surprise, and say: 'Men cannot show such skill as this. I think this doctor is helped by the angels.' The Englishman does not know that all the skill, which seems to him so wonderful, is from those first books published four thousand years ago.

"The colleges which teach the skill and knowledge of western nations, as distinguished from those of the Orient, were commenced in China about twenty years ago, and they teach all professions. Some of the teachers come from Germany, and some come from England. Their ways of teaching and their rules of management are just the same as those of colleges in America, and I need not describe them in detail. During the past three years, many states have established these colleges, and have brought citizens of western countries to be members of the different faculties. They teach all professions, and more colleges are constantly being established.

"Throughout China, however, the study of the English systems of medicine is growing less and less. The Chinese regard English physicians only as surgeons, in the doing of such operations, as removing tumors and similar external difficulties. In other matters they do not have much confidence in these doctors. Consequently the doctors do not have many patients among the native people. They prefer the medical system taught in the ancient books printed four thousand years ago."

THE HERBAL REMEDIES.

A CLASSIFICATION OF HERBAL MEDICINES.

WHENCE THEIR POWER IS DERIVED AND THEIR ACTION ON THE HUMAN BODY.

Everything in the world is included in five elements, namely: Water, mineral, vegetation, fire and earth. In the vital organs there are also five different elements, and everything in vegetation corresponds to five kinds of elements. The power which comes from the use of these elements in vegetation is the same as the power in the different vital organs. This is a theory of very great importance, and one which I am anxious for the American people to understand.

I shall explain the simpler lessons from these facts first. In things belonging to the water element the color is black, the taste is salt, and the power is of benefit to the lower organs of the human body. The herbal medicines that are of a black color and salt taste belong to the water element, and therefore have an influence upon the kidneys and the bladder, for these organs also belong to the water element. In the vegetation element the color is blue or green and the taste is sour. So herbs of a blue or green color and sour taste are allied to the vegetation element. These have a power to contract the air in the blood, and their action assists the liver and gall, because these organs belong to the vegetable element. The color of things belonging to the fire element is red, the taste is bitter, and the power from these rushes through the system. Therefore herb remedies of a red color and bitter taste are classed with the fire element and influence the heart. the heart-case and the small intestines, which belong to the fire element. The power from these herbs rushes through the upper part of the body. The color of the earth element is yellow, its taste is sweet, and the power from it is very slow. Therefore herbal remedies of a yellow color and sweet taste belong to the earth element. These can cause the circulation to go slow and make the effect of the medicines remain in the middle of the vital organs. Their effect is upon the spleen and the stomach, because the spleen and the stomach are of the earth element. In the mineral element, the color is white, the taste is hot and the power expands. So herbal medicines of a white color and a hot taste belong to the mineral element. These cause the natural heat of the body to go down through the extremities and through the outside of the skin. These influence the action of the lungs and the larger intestines, because these organs belong to the mineral element.

Mineral produces water; water produces vegetation; vegetation produces fire; fire produces earth; earth produces mineral; these make up the five elements. The earth medicine produces the air in the blood. The mineral element is stronger than the vegetation and can control it; vegetation controls the earth and the earth controls the water; water controls the fire, and the fire controls the mineral; water can stop the fire and dissolve the mineral. The earth remedies conquer poisons.

This is the simplest explanation of the relation between the herbal remedies and their effects upon the differnt vital organs. But there are other and more abstruse variations of this subject, some of which I shall explain. When, for instance, in any herb the color belongs to one element, and the taste to another, then there is a different power and a different effect from those which exist when both color and tast are to the same elment. Thus, the color may be white, belonging to the mineral element, and the taste sweet, belonging to the earth. Or the taste may be hot, belonging to the mineral, and the color green, belonging to vegetation. In this way one herb has two or more different elements in its composition. It therefore has more than one effect and more than one power.

It also happens that some medicines of black color and salt taste do not belong to the water element; some of green color and sour taste do not belong to the vegetable element; some of red color and bitter taste do not belong to the fire element; some of yellow color and sweet taste do not belong to the earth element, and some of white color and hot taste do not belong to the mineral element. This is because there are six varieties of air or currents of power in these which control, and then the taste and color lose their natural power. When the color and the taste are equal, the taste is a better guide than the color, but if the air and the taste are equal, the air is a better guide than the taste.

THE PREPARATION OF REMEDIES.

Sometimes, also, in these medicines the color is very plain, and the taste is very slight; in some the color is very indefinite, but the taste is very strong and the air is very light; in some the air is very heavy, but the taste is very slight; in some the air and taste are both strong; in some they are both light. There are many differences of this kind, but when the color and taste are equal, the taste controls the color; if the air and taste are equal, the air controls the taste; the power or effect comes from the air, and the taste loses is natural power. Every kind of herb has its own power and differs from the others, just as every man differs from all others in his personal appearance and looks. The doctors must understand this philosophy very clearly. Then when they understand about every herb medicine, and understand what kind of power each herb has, they must also understand how to join the medicines into the different combinations which are called remedies. If a few kinds of herbs are joined without much power, they cannot produce a beneficial result. They cannot conquer sickness, and cannot be called remedies. They do not benefit the patient, because they do not overcome disease. By mixing these medicines and making many changes, many different effects are produced. With some kinds of remedies the power goes through the upper part of the body; in some it goes through the lower; in some through the left side; in some through the right side, and in some through the outside of the body, or the skin; and sometimes the effect is retained in the vital organs, in the inner portions of the body, or it may go through the liver or through the kidneys.

Each of the vital organs, therefore, when it is out of sorts or sick, has its own remedy. When there is sickness in two or more of the vital organs, then there is need of more than one remedy.

ACTION OF THE REMEDIES.

Some remedies can assist only one organ; others can assist more than one. Some kinds of remedies are good for both internal and external use. Some other kinds of power go through the whole body, from the top of the head to the bottom of the foot. Some remedies can relieve excessive heat or fever and can help the system that is very weak. They can prevent sickness if taken in time or can cure sickness, even when the patient is so ill as to be nearly dead. Moreover if a remedy or prescription is very skillfully prepared, sometimes with ten or twenty different medicines, it may bring more force to all of the vital organs and to the whole body. On the other hand, certain combinations, or remedies, are so arranged that each herb loses its natural power or effect, and the whole combination, taken together, has only one effect, or only two or three different effects. If the physician does not understand exactly the variations produced by the six kinds of air or currents of power, he cannot use his skill to produce these results. The six kinds of air in the medicines respond to six kinds through the system of the patient; but there are still another six kinds of air in the atmosphere, which are different from these. The explanation of this is very difficult and abstruse. It would require a book of about 80,000 words and is altogether too long to be discussed here. We shall hereafter write such a book and shall tell about the power of the medicines, how that power is obtained and what its effects are on the human system. From the more than two thousand kinds of medicines we shall search out and condense the more than four hundred kinds that are essential and best for the white man to use.

VIVISECTION AMONG THE CHINESE.

HOW THE EARLY PHYSICIANS OF CHINA WHO WERE ALSO EMPERORS EMPLOYED CRIMINALS FOR THE BENEFIT OF SCIENCE.

THE TRUE HISTORY OF AN IMPORTANT AND MUCH DISCUSSED SUBJECT. A SHORT ROUTE TO EXACT KNOWLEDGE OF THE HUMAN BODY AND ITS FUNCTIONS---RESULTS WHICH HAVE JUSTIFIED THE COST.

Judge Philip Thier, of Berkeley, is a warm friend of the Chinese system of medicine, having been cured of kidney troubles by this system, and his wife having been cured of dropsy. In an interview a few weeks ago, he remarked: "When I was in China, I heard something said about the use of vivisection many years ago in establishing the principles of the Chinese system of medicine and anatomy. It was said that the early doctors employed criminals condemned to death for this purpose. Can you tell me something about the details of this practice, whatever it may have been?"

The reply to this inquiry was as follows: "Yes, there was something of that kind in China, many years ago, when the first 'holy men' received a great power in healing from the God. But it seems that all of this cannot be understood by the common thought and I am afraid that the subject is too new for Americans to understand, and it is contrary to their ideas of what is right and proper." But Judge Thier answered: "No, vivisection has been advocated by great physicians in Europe, who have desired to practice it there, but have been forbidden by their governments. But it is certainly better to study anatomy on the live body than on the dead body, at least you will get better results in this way. Everybody admits that, and I think it would be proper for you to tell something about the practice of vivisection among the Chinese." So we have given the following account of this very ancient custom:

Criminals condemned to capital punishment furnished the subjects for vivisection, which practice gave the Chinese their first knowledge of anatomy and of the action of remedies. The history of this practice may be considered in two ways; first, as related to the use of the herbal remedies, and second, as related to the study of anatomy. When Chinese medicine was reduced to a system, many hundred years ago, capital punishment was much more frequent than it is today, just as it was more frequent in England, and even in America, some hundreds of years ago, than it is now, and there were therefore many more criminals condemned to death who could be used for this purpose. The first "holy men" in China, who were wonderful physicians used capital punishment to try their herbal remedies; and the second "holy men," who were wonderful physicians, used it for the study of anatomy. I shall tell you first about trying the herbal remedies by means of men who were condemned to death.

This was four thousand years ago, and was the commencement of medical knowledge among the Chinese. The name of the first "holy man" who was a wonderful physician was Son Non. He commenced his work by finding out the cereals that were useful for the people as food. Afterwards he studied all forms of vegetation, and then thought that he ought to commence to treat diseases. He had learned more plainly than anybody else that everything in the world is included in five kinds of elements. He divided these five natural elements into water, vegetation, fire, earth and mineral. All herbal medicines are chosen and classified according to their relations to these five natural elements.

Some kinds of vegetation, however, are very poisonous. Some kinds are not at all poisonous. And some kinds are a little poisonous, but their poison may be taken away by using certain liquids. But everything in vegetation had to be chewed or drank before its nature was known. So, every day, Son Non tested the herbal medicines in order to teach students who were learning from him. Some days he tried poisonous herbs, and three times he appeared to be dead from the use of these, but the students used a certain liquid preparation that he had ready, and saved his life three times. His genuine book is "Poon Chow Kien," and there is proof in his first book of these facts. He says: "Three times he tried the poison herbs and made himself as if dead and was saved by the liquid." Every student tried to take care of his teacher and asked him to permit him to try the poisonous herbs in his stead.

故事在本經載神農嘗百草
一日三死三甦

Then Son Non said: "No. Because God has given me extraordinary power and wisdom to study the herbal medicines and to treat sickness, and that is my mission in life. It is not good for me to let some other people do this." Then the student would say: "It is true that God has given you extraordinary powers. Then it must be necessary for you to learn thoroughly. And if you try the poisonous herbs and they kill you, then we cannot find one more man in the world with the same purpose that you have. Then this system of medicine will be only one-half done, and this kind of skill will be broken down. Then the world will lose a great benefit. But if you permit us to learn what kinds of herbs are poisonous and to get acquainted with them, and then use some other medicines to take away the poisons, then you may try them, and at the same time you may take care of your life. In this way you can keep your health, and at the same time find out about the poisonous herbs. Then this kind of skill will be understood and that part of the book will be done. This is the best way. But if we try the poison, and it makes us die, then you can make an examination, and you will know how our lives were lost. And even if, unfortunately, one of us should die, still your studies will not be broken down when half completed."

Son Non, however, would not permit the student to try the poisons and next day he himself tried them again. He tried some kind of a poison which made his tongue and throat swell, and he was nearly dead. But he used a liquid, which made him better. Still, he was

四千年前內經第一本第一則

黃帝內經素問卷之一

錢塘張志聰隱菴集註
同學莫承藝仲超叅訂
門人朱景韓濟公校正

上古天真論篇第一
　上古謂所生之來天真天乙始生之真元也
　首四篇論調精神氣血所生之來謂之精故
　首論精兩精相搏謂之神故次論
　神氣乃精水中之生陽故後論氣

昔在黃帝生而神靈弱而能言幼而徇齊長而敦敏
成而登天狗音循長上聲〇按史記黃帝姓公孫名
軒轅有熊國君少典之子繼神農氏而有

The above is a fac-simile of the fire page of the oldest book extant treating of Chinese medicine, written 4000 years ago. This very weak, and for a few days was unable to do any work. Then all the students went to tell the Emperor. And the Emperor called togther his ministers, and tried to find out a good way to try these herbs. Some of the ministers said that it would be a good plan to use the criminals condemned to capital punishment, and to try the poisonous medicines with them; and they sent for Son Non and laid the plan before him.

Then Son Non said: "I do not want to compel the criminals to do that for me. Tomorrow have all of the condemned meet together, and if they are very willing to help me, let them raise their hands. If more than half raise their hands, then I shall be very glad to follow that plan." So the next day this was done, and all of the condemned raised up their hands, and all said: "We are very glad to do that, and to give up our lives to help you." Then, after that, everything went well; and Son Non finished his book. And a law was passed to the effect that no poisons should be used internally for medicine. But doctors were permitted to use poisons externally for diseases like cancer, ringworm, tumors, piles, etc. In ringworm, for instance, the disease comes from a little microbe, and it was lawful to use poisons to destroy them. After the microbe has been killed by using strong external remedies, then strong medicine must be used to draw out the poison which is the effect of these remedies. After the poisoned water has run out, gentle remedies are used to heal the flesh and make the cure complete.

From that time there has been great benefit to the world from Son Non's book and many diseases have been cured, so that this benefit has gone all through the world. And Son Non's merit was so great that the whole nation honored him, and, after the Emperor died, the people chose Son Non to be Emperor. During his reign he formed the character "Yeok," which means medicine. This character is composed of three different words. The word at the top means grass; that in the middle means happy or fortunate, and that at the foot means tree. The adding of new words to the Chinese language, at that time, was a prerogative of the Emperor.

At this time only herbal remedies were permitted to be used, according to the law on this subject, and nothing whatever from the animal or mineral kingdoms. But afterwards there were many different schools of physicians. Some of these wanted to use sharp-pointed tubes, by which they perforated the skin and made the blood run, an operation similar to the cupping of American physicians, and there were many other different forms of treatment. Some doctors wanted to use the knife, and some wanted to sear the flesh by hot irons and by other uses of fire, burning the pores of the skin in different ways. Some wanted to use a remedy called "Li." in connection with thin slices of ginger root. The "Li" looks like cotton. The thin strips of ginger would be laid upon the skin and the "Li" burned over this, the intention being to have the fire go through the pores. The ginger, being wet, would prevent it from burning too deeply, and would cause it to burn slowly. This was to be kept up as long as the patient could stand it, and then taken away. It was applied at first only warm, then hotter and finally as hot as it could be endured, after which it was taken away. There were all these and other different kinds of skill and treatment. But the people seemed to be afraid of the dangers of these methods, and the doctors who tried to cure in this way did not have very much business, and there were only a few students who learned these ways.

Besides these there were other doctors who used plasters only, and some used liniments; but these doctors did not understand how to remove the root of the diseases, which is internal. So the people were not satisfied with them. Other doctors used materials from animals, and mixed them with the herbal remedies. Some used minerals with the herbs, but the educated people were not satisfid with them and liked the pure herbs better. After a few hundred years an Emperor passed a law to stop the use of anything of this sort by physicians, and to prevent such physicians from practicing; and requiring all doctors to use the pure herbs, and also to pass an examination at the Imperial Medical College. After passing this examination, they were allowed to practice. But after this law had been in force several centuries, the Chinese nation grew so large and the population was so great that there were not enough doctors capable of passing this examination, which was very hard, and could only be passed after a long course of study; so that there were not enough doctors furnished to take care of all the people. Then the law was broken down, and any one was permitted to be a doctor if he wanted to be, and every man or woman was permitted to use his or her own free will in selecting a doctor. Still the physician to the Emperor must pass an examination. The law was not changed in this respect.

After listening to this account, Judge Thier said: "I am very much pleased, indeed, to hear this account of vivisection and of the origin of medicine among the Chinese and its history. But I would still like to know something about the history of anatomy." In reply to this we have prepared the following account:

The second "holy man" who was a wonderful physician was named Hin Yuen, and the people called him Wong Ti. He wrote two different series of books. One series was called "Ling Soo Keng," and the other series was called "Soo Mon Keng." The first pages of the "Soo Mon Keng" contain a few words in reference to Wong Ti, to show that he was surely a "holy man," and saying: "He is wise and his wisdom cannot be comprehended by common thought."

When Wong Ti was born, the very day of his birth, he was very smart and could talk with his mother at once in a way that was very wonderful. The people heard of this, and were very much surprised at such an instance, and came to see him. They thought him very remarkable, and everybody said: "That boy has great wisdom from God. God has permitted very great wisdom to come to him. By and by he will surely be something wonderful and of great benefit to the world." After Wong Ti had grown to be a great man, he established the principles of the five relations, as follows: First, as between sovereigns and ministers; second, as between parents and children; third, as between brothers and sisters; fourth, as between husband and wife; and fifth, as between friends. The principles of these he laid down, and they became very celebrated in a book of philosophy. He also liked to study the works of Son Non on treating the diseases of the people.

After Son Non died, Wong Ti was chosen for Emperor. During his reign he discovered a wonderful man, whose name was Kay Bak, who had helped the Emperor in preparing his works an anatomy. When he commenced this series of books he made use of the criminals who were condemned to capital punishment. He first gave the criminal who was to be used, medicine for a few months. Then he gave him a liquid, something like ether or chloroform, which acted as an anaesthetic. He then performed an operation by which he could observe all the functions of the body and its vital organs. He had a device by which the interior of the human body could be lighted up so that everything could be seen. He discovered the twelve different vital organs within the body and the twelve pulses which go through the body to the outside. It is very hard for the unskilled to distinguish these twelve different pulses. But if a physician is well educated in this respect and has had a good teacher to teach him, then, from the pulses of the outside of the body, he can understand the condition of the interior organs and of the vital functions, whether they are sick or are in good health.

I will give you an illustration of this. If there are many pumpkins growing in a piece of ground, crowded together within a little space, after they have grown up, all the extremeties and leaves spread very widely over the ground, and any one who looks will find it hard to tell which stem belongs to any given root. But if there are stems of different colors from two different roots, then you can trace one color from the stems and the leaves to the root to which they belong. In this way you can find all of the stems that belong to some one root.

In the same way the students of Chinese medicine are taught to understand all of the vital organs and what kind of power comes from each of them, and what natural taste and color belongs to them, and also how some kinds of medicine bring out the natural color from the different vital organs. The students must understand what elements belong to the vital organs, and then find out the five different kinds of elements in the herbs which benefit the five classes of vital organs. But the people thought this a very curious thing, and did not understand it at all. So I will give you an easy way to know about it. In the vegetation element, the natural color is green. Now the gall liquid and the natural juices which pass from the liver are green. So you may know that the liver and the gall belong to the vegetation element. And this further fact is an additional proof of this. In some people the gall liquid is yellow. But if you have the proper medicine to bring out the natural color, then you will find the green mingled with the yellow. Again, the naturel color of the fire element is red. Now the heart controls the actions of the blood of the body, through the heart-case and the arteries. The blood is red. Therefore the heart and the heart-case belong to the fire element. The natural taste of the water element is salt. The bladder gets its power from the kidneys and turns all of the liquids of the body into urine, the taste of which is salt. From this you may know that the kidneys and the bladder belong to the water element. The natural color of the earth element is yellow. The stomach gets power from the spleen, which produces the gastric juice. The color in this case is yellow, and if the same element is found in the passages you will find that the color is yellow; and so you can know that the spleen and stomach belong to the earth element. The

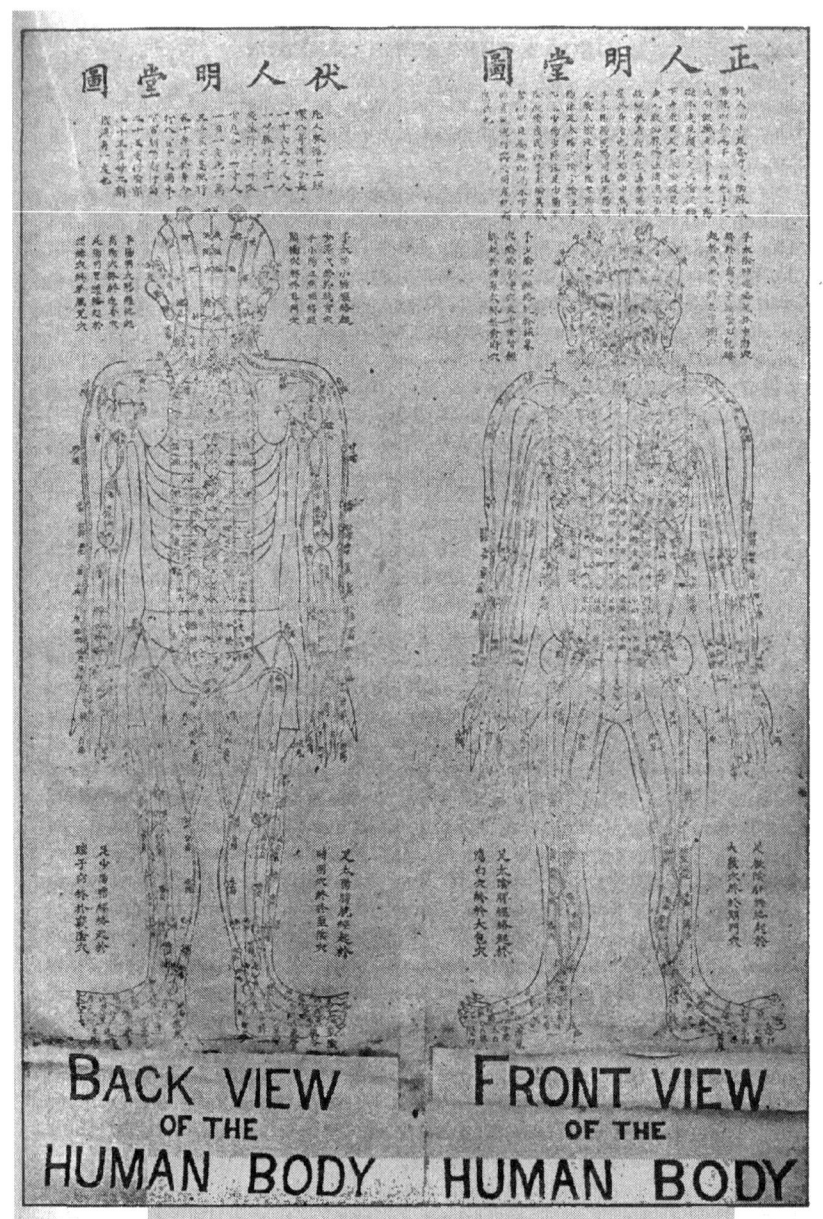

CHART SHOWING THE TWELVE PULSE OF THE HUMAN BODY.

color of the natural element in minerals is white, and the color of the lungs is also white. From this we know that the lungs belong to the mineral element.

An experiment to show this may be made by cooking the lungs of a hog in boiling water. First the lungs should be cleaned and all the blood taken away, so as to show it in its natural state. Use boiling water to cook it, for an hour, and you will then find that it is white. If you cook the stomach in the same way you will find that is white, too, but a little bit yellow, because the stomach partakes of two different elements. If you cook other organs you will find the color different, because the elements are different. What I am defining now applies to the anatomy of well people. In another way the anatomy of sick people will show what conditions sickness within the body brings. Different illnesses make different conditions.

The early investigators killed different men, and found out about all these things. They took criminals who were sick and cured them. Then they killed them and cut them open to show what benefits had been received from the different kinds of treatment and how the conditions had been changed. To make another test they took well people and experimented to find what herbs would injure them. After they had given medicines, the effects of which they could not cure, they studied the results and what injuries had been received from these medicines. Then, after awhile, they came to the point where they made no more mistakes, and where they had learned about the action of all the remedies. Then they showed all of these to the people. Then they took well people and tried some poisonous medicines, afterwards using medicines to cure the effects of these and proving to the people the benefit that had been received. And they explained very clearly all that they had learned in reference to anatomy. The work known as "Ling Soo Keng" is composed of nine volumes, and the work "Soo Mon Keng" is composed of nine volumes also. Each book filled a complete house, because, at that time, they had no paper, but the books were written on bamboo slips with bamboo brushes and using the sap of some kinds of plants for ink. And, because the reasoning was very deep, and hard to be condensed into short words, they could not put all into the books, but taught the students by word of mouth. Since that time there have been plenty of teachers, and students, the students becoming teachers in their turn.

When the work was completed there were still plenty of criminals condemned to capital punishment waiting to be used in the interests of the study of anatomy. But Wong Ti said: "The book is done. We need not kill any more criminals." Then they opened the jails and pardoned those who were waiting there, and gave them their lives. "And all the people were so glad that they made a big noise and laughed like the sound of an earthquake."

After hearing this account, Judge Thier remarked: "This is also certainly very wonderful, and I have been greatly interested in hearing this history. Some people may not understand all of this, and may not believe. But the best way is to keep this account and to think it over. We shall surely find in it some very wonderful lessons. Some of these things are pretty deep, and we probably will not understand them at once. But if we reflect upon them we shall find a great deal that we may understand and that will make the philosophy of the Chinese system of medicine clearer to us. And I am very much obliged to you for telling us all about these matters."

CHAPTER VII.

THE DISEASES OF WOMEN.

THEIR TREATMENT BY THE HERBAL REMEDIES—THE MOST RATIONAL AND SUCCESSFUL METHOD KNOWN.

The diseases of women are among the most common and the most formidable of the maladies with which the physician of the present day has to contend. The causes of these diseases are very numerous. It would be impossible and is unnecessary to attempt to enumerate them all. Modern ways of life are responsible for most of them, high living, rich foods, late hours, parties, balls, demands of society and excitements of all kinds. Overwork is frequently an exciting cause; anxiety is another. Various perversions of marriage attempts to prevent child-birth, and ignorance, carelessness or lack of care during and after child-birth. All of these causes, and others, are constantly at work. Many women doubtless have an inherited predisposition to these diseases, and many young women acquire a predisposition through overwork at school, or through early efforts at earning a livelihood. Whatever is a shock to the nervous system or whatever overtaxes it is a cause as well as those causes, such as a miscarriage, which have a direct effect.

The Chinese system of medicine is particularly adapted to the treatment of these diseases. Its great variety of harmless, efficient herbs come into play in every phase of these diseases. If the trouble depends upon mal-nutrition and a degenerate condition of the nerves the Chinese have special herb foods, which supply the needed elements. If the disorder arises from an impure or disordered state of the blood, this system has many remedies which cleanse and enrich the blood, enabling it to have healing effect and an upbuilding effect as well. These disorders are invariably accompanied by fever or inflammation in some part of the patient's body, and the Chinese remedies to reduce and prevent inflammation are very numerous and very effective. Those cases even in which the American physician has no remedy except the knife, yield rapidly to the herbal treatment.

In China medicine and surgery are distinct professions, and the two are not usually followed by the same physician. But medicine attempts and accomplishes many things which American physicians turn over to the surgeons. This is seen in the treatment of many diseases of the bones, which, in America, are treated by mechanical supports, by scraping of the bone and other operations or by amputation. The Chinese doctor cures these cases by medicines alone, perhaps aided, in some instances, by the use of plasters and linaments, where there is impure blood or other poisonous liquids to be drawn away. The Chinese think it is just as easy to feed a bone as it is to feed a muscle. One can be made to grow as well as the other. Both have circulation and are nourished by the blood. The only difference is that a longer time is usually required to strengthen a weakened bone by feeding it than to strengthen a weakened muscle, because its substance is harder and its circulation slower. A change, therefore, requires a greater length of time, but it is just as certain in the one case as in the other.

The same reasoning applies to abnormal growths in the womb or ovaries, or to ulcerations, enlargements of the tissues or of the substance of the womb, cancers, tumors and similar difficulites. These things can all be checked and cured by internal medication much easier than by mechanical means, by scraping and cutting, or by amputation. Surgical operations never accomplish a cure. They simply take away something from the body and maim it in one way or another. When a physician recommends a surgical operation he admits that the means at his command are insufficient, that he hasn't the remedies to meet the case, and this is, in fact, the reason that so many surgeons flourish upon the disorders of women, and find in them their broadest yet constantly growing field. Doctors lack the remedies to meet the need, and as they haven't got them, they cannot prescribe them.

Let us consider in greater detail some of the more prevalent forms of the diseases of women and see how the Chinese system of medicine is particularly adapted to cure them. Derangements of the menstrual function are among the most common and the most injurious. The menstrual function in a normal woman ought to be practically painless, instead of a source of misery and illness as it often is. Its perversion takes a score of forms; sometimes it is delayed, sometimes premature, sometimes scanty, sometimes profuse and often accompanied by severe headaches, bearing-down pains, and even by hysteria and complete exhaustion. It is usually functional, that is, depending upon defects in circulation, impairment of the nervous system, or a generally debilitated condition, but it may come from an enlarged or ulcerated condition of the womb, or other local causes.

In either case the herbal remedies act efficiently and promptly. A tonic medicine is not what is needed, because, if there is inflammation, as there usually is, a tonic is simply an addition of fuel to a fire already existing. Neither are local applications of any permanent value. They may relieve the local pain for a time, and may be of some transient benefit by toning up the organs involved, as by use of electricity; but the beneficial effect soon passes; the original causes are still at work, and the original results come back again. Suppressed or painful menstruation is often a result of a cold, and the physician usually thinks that if the menses can be brought on again, a cure is accomplished, not stopping to think that the poisonous conditions which resulted from the cold and caused the suppression in the first place still remain in the system and are liable to produce the same effect again. Sometimes there is an unnatural contraction of the mouth of the womb, closing it, and some sort of an operation which forces it open is thought necessary in order to permit a resumption of the menstrual flow.

These ideas are all wrong. What is needed, nine time out of ten, is a general cleansing of the system and a restoration of the normal activity of all the bodily functions. If poisons have accumulated in the blood through a failure of the bowels, the kidneys and the skin to do their work properly, this difficulty must be removed before they can be any permanent improvement. If the stomach does not act perfectly, and there is consequently a lack of nutriment for the nerves and the muscles and a thinning of the blood, then that organ and its assistant organs of digestion must be compelled to perform their functions as nature intended. If poison has been left in the system through a cold which has settled in the womb and the ovaries and clogs their action, that poison must be removed and the trouble will be cured. Local applications are almost always useless, except, perhaps to a certain extent in connection with internal treatment. The healthful performance of the menstrual function is only accomplished in a healthful state of the whole body, and that must be brought about before there can be any definite and constant improvement.

The same facts apply to the period known as "the change of life," which is a period of great pain and danger for many women. Some women take eight or ten years to pass through this transition, which ought to be accomplished in two or three at the farthest, and without undue inconveniences or suffering. The woman who enters upon this period with all her bodily functions in a normal condition has nothing to fear; nature takes care of the rest. But the woman who commences it with digestion, nutrition, elimination and circulation all wrong, with the stomach, kidneys, liver, bowels all slow or imperfect in doing their work, must expect trouble, as a matter of course. And this is too often the case, owing to American ways of life, which regard the pleasures of the table and the excitements of society as of greater importance than health.

Falling of the womb is another difficulty which too often receives only illogical and patch-work treatment. The muscles supporting the womb in place become relaxed, through a general debilitated condition of the system, or from some local strain or injury, or the womb becomes thickened or enlarged through various causes. The usual treatment is to attempt to support the organ in place by a mechanical device, such as a rubber ring or pessary, when the muscles are weakened; or to cut away a portion by "curetting" or scraping the parts most accessible, thus trying to reduce it in size and weight, and various injections and suppositories are used with the hope of strengthening the muscles and causing them to hold the organ in its proper place. The failure of all of these methods arises from the fact that that the original causes are still at work, except when the injury comes from some sudden strain, such as attempting to lift too great a weight or from some similar cause. Unless those causes can be permanently removed there can be no permanent improvement.

Ulcerous growths in the womb or vagina, cancers of the womb and similar conditions, which take the forms of ulcers, of greater or less severity and danger, and such diseases as leuchorrea are also usually treated by local applications, by antiseptic injections, suppositories and other devices to introduce various medications, which are supposed to heal the diseased surfaces. Cancer of the breast is a sympathetic complication to which the same reasoning applies. All of these troubles depend upon some remote cause, some functional derangement, or some poison in the system, often left there by lack of care in child-birth or by miscarriage, but sometimes coming from a cause that is only indirectly connected with the menstrual function or the generative organs. There is no cure, because this source of poisonous accumulation, whatever it may be, is not removed, and, while the local treatment may render temporary relief, it cannot remove the disturbing cause because it is not directed against that cause.

Now the herbal remedies assist nature in these cases, as in all others, in two ways. They purify and enrich the blood, and they furnish foods for the nourishment of different portions of the body. These two facts are beyond dispute; everybody can understand them. We derive our daily food from the animal and vegetable kingdoms, but there is no mineral substance that anybody ever takes for food, or that will permanently strengthen the system. In the same way we may find vegetable substances which are special foods for the different organs of the body, and have a direct and healthful influence upon them.

Now compare the use of these substances as medicines with the use of minerals or local applications or mechanical devices. We can understand how a vegetable substance which is in the nature of a food can be taken into the blood and carried to the weakened portion of the body which needs special feeding and will there render the necessary assistance. But we cannot understand anything of the sort in reference to a mineral which is indigestible, or to a poison, which is injurious to a well person. Here is the whole difference in the methods of treatment in a nutshell. After these points are established and everybody will admit them, successful treatment by herbal remedies is simply a matter of knowing which are beneficial under the conditions of each case. This special knowledge the Chinese have been acquiring for the past four thousand years by the exclusive use of these remedies in their practice of medicine.

Under this view of the case, which certainly must appeal to the common sense of every reader who will take the trouble to think for himself, is not at least advisable for the suffering woman to make a test of these remedies before submitting to an operation or despairing utterly of ever obtaining relief? There is no need of any humbug or secrecy or false modesty about these matters. And there is no need of being frightened half to death over a case that may not be as bad as the sufferer thinks it to be. A particularly wretched accompaniment of many of these cases is the melancholia or despondency accompanying them. The inevitable depression of the nervous system makes the victim to these troubles believe that there can be no help for her, while the truth may be that a comparatively short and simple course of treatment will restore her completely to health. The effort is certainly well worth the making.

There are hundreds of cases on record in which the diseases of women have been perfectly and permanently cured by the Chinese herbal remedies.

Several years ago Dr. J. A. Shesler, an American physician residing in San Jose, California, reported a case where a tumor that was estimated to weigh thirty pounds was removed from a woman by a Chinese physician through the use of internal remedies alone. In other words it was absorbed into the blood and carried away. There are cases which form a part of the judicial records of the State of California in which women have testified to similar cures upon the witness stand and under oath.

Of course, a cure of this sort requires time. Such a thing cannot be accomplished in a day except by very violent means. The herbal remedies are the opposite of violent. Their action is gradual and accumulative, that is, the good they do in one day is added to that of the day before, and the favorable effect is kept up until a cure is accomplished. If women would employ these remedies at the commencement of their ailments instead, of as at present, after they have progressed for a long time, a vast amount of suffering would be spared them.

TESTIMONIALS.

We Offer the Following Testimonials from Ladies Who Have Used Our Remedies.

Mrs. Gertrude E. Samo of Los Angeles, writes:

The Foo and Wing Herb Company—Gentlemen: I take great pleasure in complying with your request for a few lines for the book you are compiling for the benefit of the sick.

As you have done so much for me, I am anxious to do all I can for suffering humanity. My illness commenced in Washington, D.C., where I lived for over twenty years, and having several deaths in my family, who were attended by some of the most noted physicians of the city, I felt I must obey when my doctor said I would be subject to gastric fever if I remained there, so I moved to Riverside, Cal., ten years ago. I was very well for several years, but was then again attacked and for six years I was a confirmed invalid with chronic diarrhea and other troubles. I think I would have been paralyzed by this time if I had not met with Dr. Foo, for our own physicians only relieved me for a time and could not cure me. I saw Dr. Foo's advertisement in The Times of Los Angeles, diagnosing by the pulse, and went to him without knowing any one he had cured, and when he diagnosed my case by my pulse, without any question except my age, and told me how I was affected so accurately, and the cause, and that it was of long standing, I was astonished and convinced that he knew what to do for me, and commenced treatment at once, and took a large cup of the herb tea, to the horror of my daughter, who had nursed me so long and was so careful of what I ate and drank. I told her that I felt I was guided by a heavenly Power, and that I was acting wisely of which I am now fully convinced. I took treatment two weeks before he could tell if he could cure me. He found he could, having controlled my bowels from the first dose, telling just what the herb tea would do. It was marvelous to me, after being treated six years by our physicians. He said it would take at least six months, taking two courses of medicine. I improved all the time, and then, at his advice, left off four months, and am now taking treatment a short time longer, as he recommended it. I have great confidence in him, and am thoroughly satisfied with his treatment. He is an honorable, humane, gentlemanly man, and would compare favorably with cultivated men from any part of the globe. There is no question as regards his scientific ability against an understanding of the condition of any patient through the pulse alone. His methods of examination are truly refined. I have conversed with many of Dr. Foo's patients and find that they lose the prejudice as they become better acquainted with him and see more clearly the evidences of his skill. So strongly am I impressed with this fact, that I wonder why our American physicians do not adopt some of these methods, or at least, investigate them in a fair and candid spirit.

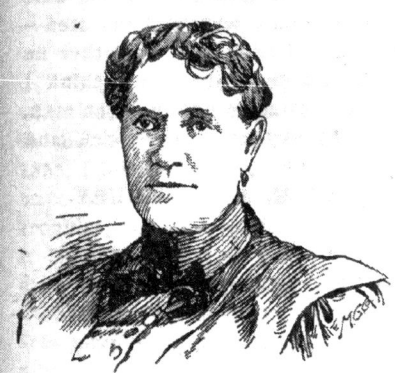

MRS. GERTRUDE R. SAMO.

In the matter of diet, Dr. Foo shows great skill and study. You are not allowed to find out for yourself (as I formerly had, to my sorrow,) what is best for you to eat, as a bill of fare is provided.

Some people may think his charges for the herbs are high, but compared with the results, they are insignificant.

Hoping that these few lines will induce many who are suffering to take your treatment and be cured, I remain gratefully your friend, MRS. GERTRUDE SAMO,

1818 E. Second street, corner Boyle avenue.

The following letter from a former well-known resident of Redlands, was addressed to a gentleman in San Bernardino, who wrote to her, making some inquiries:

LAKEWOOD, New Jersey, March 23, 1897.

Mr. F. F. Cross, San Bernardino, Cal.

Dear Sir: Your letter was forwarded to me in New York City and from there to New Jersey, where I am staying for a few weeks. I received it today, and take pleasure in saying that Dr. Foo did a great deal for me. I was suffering from biliousness and sick headache in its worst for, not being able to sit up for three days after a severe attack. I had these headaches so often that I was in a weak and feeble condition most of the time. I am thankful to say I have not had one in more than two years; it is nearer three years. I have great confidence in Dr. Foo, and think he will help you if any one can.

I consider my cure permanent. I took his treatment about nine months. It is expensive, but I think the money was well invested—not being young it took longer to cure me. I cannot tell whether he cures all cases he accepts. If he says he can cure you I think I would let him try. I consider Dr. Foo to be an honest, upright man, and would recommend him to you or to anyone who is sick and suffering, Very truly yours,

MRS. M. A. KINGSBURY.

ABSCESS OF THE WOMB AND BOWELS CURED.

LOS ANGELES, Cal., Sept. 4, 1898.

T. Foo Yuen of the Foo and Wing Herb Co.:

For the benefit of the sick and afflicted, I consider it my duty to give them my experiences of sickness and suffering, of the past twenty years. I have been doctoring with some of what are considered the best physicians both in the East and here in California. The general verdict being spleen and liver trouble. But I had no relief whatever until I began taking medicine of Dr. Foo. After diagnosing my case, he explained to my perfect satisfaction that my head trouble, stomach trouble, and severe cough, were caused by abcesses on the liver, and in the bowels and womb, leaving me in such a state that all my friends and my husband despaired of my ever getting well. At first the discharge of blood and matter from the bowels was terrible. Now the discharge has disappeared, my cough has left me, (and I did, at the time I went to Dr. Foo cough all day and all night, and had for nearly one year.) The pain in side, bloating, weakness of heart, nervousness and other troubles have left me, and I am getting stronger all the time. I am now 62 years old, and feeling better than I have for the past 25 years. Thanks be to Dr. Foo. I realize the truth more and more every day—that he has been the means of saving my life, and may he live long to help others as he has me, is my earnest wish.

Any one wishing to know the truth of this statement, can call at 1933 East Second street, Boyle Heights, and I will gladly explain all to them. MRS. A. W. SWAIN.

Mrs. W. J. Anderson of North Fair Oaks ave., Pasadena, writes:

"PASADENA, Cal., July 13, 1897.

"I had been afflicted with a complication of diseases for a number of years, and had been treated by some of the best physicians both in the East and in California, but gradually grew worse. In August, 1895, I heard of Dr. T. Foo Yuen, and decided to call on him. He at once told me of all my past, and, at that time present physical troubles, without asking me any questions whatever, and said that, if I would take his herbal remedies under his direction, they would cure me. I very reluctantly consented to try them, and must say that their effects from the first were wonderful. I continued the treatment for about seven months, all the time in doubts as to whether my improvement would be permanent, but it is now over a year since I have taken any treatment whatever, and I have been improving gradually and continually."

The following is from Mrs. T. D. Merryman of Los Angeles:

The Foo and Wing Herb Co.,

Gentlemen: It gives me great pleasure to say that your treatment in my case has been most wonderful. For over 20 years I had been an invalid and so many times had I been prostrated with inflammation of the stomach that my friends and neighbors had despaired of my life, and it seemed like an impossibility for me to rally. The February after the World's Fair I had a very severe attack of acute rheumatism. Our home physician was called in and he gave me remedies that soon brought relief, and with the aid of canes, I commenced walking a little around the house in three or four weeks. I was looking forward to a speedy recovery, but, alas! I was doomed to disappointment. I began to notice a numbness and bloating in my feet and limbs. I did not worry much about this at first, thinking that I would soon find some remedy to overcome and ward off the disease, believing it to be

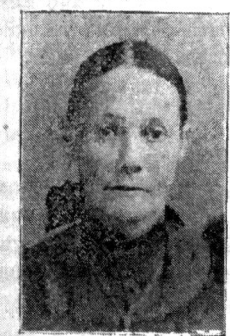

MRS. T. D. MERRYMAN.

just common dropsy. I used the very best medicines I knew of but all of this was of no avail. I then went to the Hot Springs at San Jacinto, taking hot mud baths, as my friends thought they would certainly bring relief, but the bloating kept increasing. I then felt alarmed and called our physician. He then told me that I was in a very critical condition, and unless I could get help very soon I would not last very long. He told me he had only one remedy to offer, and said he believed it would help me; if it did not then he could no nothing more for me. I took the remedy about four months and was very much better, so that I had hopes of regaining my health. Last fall, however, after all the medicine I had taken, the bloating again increased. I sent away and got more of the medicine and used it the same as before, but this time with no success. I then called another physician, but I gradually grew weaker and more helpless—so feeble that I could scarcely move around the house. About this time there appeared a letter in the Los Angeles Times concerning T. Foo Yuen. I read it; then other letters appeared telling of his success in curing some almost incurable diseases. These I read also. I visited him, and he told me, after examination of the pulse, without any questioning, more accurately than I could have told myself, and I felt confident that he thoroughly understood my case. He showed so much interest in me that I felt I could not make a mistake by placing myself under his treatment, which I did on the 22nd of last February. I feel today that I am a perfectly changed being. I can easily walk half a mile to church, while before I could not walk half a block without suffering.

I can truly say I will heartily recommend all my friends and any that may need medical aid to T. Foo Yuen, 903 South Olive, Los Angeles, Cal. MRS. T. D. MERRYMAN.
3020 Hoover street, Los Angeles, Cal., September 4, 1896.

The following letter, which was originally printed in the Los Angeles Times at a time when there was some newspaper discussion over the Chinese methods of practice, is from a lady, who, although for many years an invalid, is well known as a contributor to various periodicals of Southern California. The letter explains itself:

BLUFF HOUSE, ALHAMBRA, Cal., Jan. 19, 1896.

To the Editor of The Times:

In view of the really malignant attacks now being made on a quiet, educated gentleman, T. Foo Yuen, and stirred with the sympathy of a long suffering, sorely-tried invalid for my confreres in misfortune, I take the liberty of begging that you will give this space in your publication. It is well known that I have been a hopeless invalid for twenty-three years, gradually growing worse with excruciating suffering from head to foot that took various forms, each more torturing than the others, and finally resulting in complete helplessness and a wheel chair. During the twenty-three years I have consulted the best physicians in New York, San Francisco and Los Angeles. I have found many conscientious gentlemen and kindly friends among the number, but none who could cure even one of my manifold torments and only two who have ever given me temporary relief—one physician in New York and the other in Los Angeles, who relieved me of eczema, but said frankly that he could not cure it under my condition of helplessness. Last November I consulted Dr. T. Foo Yuen, and he gave me quite a different diagnosis from any former physician—a diagnosis that many facts and long experience thoroughly confirmed. As I am a mere "stranded wreck upon the shores of time," Dr. Foo Yuen does not promise me an entire set of "clearance papers;" but he gives me hopes of a better ending to a disastrous voyage—what no other physician has ever done; hopes that are being verified in this much, viz.: Since the short time in which I have taken his very cleanly medicinal herbs I have been entirely freed from a most atrocious eczema of nearly six years' standing, that if Dante had ever experienced for one month, he would have added it to his list of other delights in his "Inferno;" and a dropsical affection causing difficulty in breathing, blurred vision, heaviness of head, and dullness of hearing. If he does as much for me in the next three months, life will, at least, possess a portion of its old-time charm. It seems to me that some of my spindle-shanked, blue-lipped countrymen would better try and emulate the fresh-lipped, physical condition of Dr. T. Foo Yuen themselves, before dictating to others. As an earnest advocate of square-bound, even-handed justice to all men, whether of the Occident or the Orient, I wish to give honor where honor is due. Now, Mr. Editor, in view of these few simple facts, and I am not alone, I ask, is it manly, is it even decent for presumably fair-minded men to wage war by falsification and otherwise on their suffering kind? Since it is we the "rejected invalids" whom they prosecute under the tenuous guise of "protecting the invalid." As if physical suffering, pre-supposed idiocy and the need of a guardian. I have always found T. Foo Yuen a kindly, courteous gentleman in all my dealings with him, and his system of medication pre-eminently dainty, cleanly and efficacious. EMILY GRAY MAYBERRY.

LETTER FROM MRS. ELIZA A. OTIS.

The following general letter of commendation of T. Foo Yuen's skill and methods seems to find its most appropriate place here. It is from Mrs. Eliza A. Otis, a talented writer, and well known in California. She is the wife of Brigadier-General Harrison Gray Otis, editor of the Los Angeles Times, a man of national reputation, at one time in command of a division of the United States troops at Manila. Mrs. Otis says:

"I have had the pleasure of a brief acquaintance with Dr. Tom Foo Yuen and have found him to be not only an agreeable and cultivated gentleman, but one well versed in the medical science of his country, and with a large knowledge of medical herbs and their proper use."

1948 Grand Avenue.

A BRIEF BUT VIVID STATEMENT.

No. 1609 Atlantic Avenue.

ATLANTIC CITY, N. J., Nov. 26, 1896.

Dear Doctor: I feel that I ought to give you a testimonial of what you have done for me. When I called on you I was suffering with a bad cough, thought I had consumption. In five days your medicine cured my cough. I was also suffering from diabetes, was poisoned inside and outside, my hands were in a deadful state, swollen out of shape. I was compelled to keep my fingers bound up. Nothing seemed to relieve me. My family doctor said it was diabetic trouble. I also took a course of treatment from a specialist in New York, but without relief.

Thank God, all is now over. I am 65 years of age, and reside at Atlantic City, N. J. Respectfully, MRS. E. L. SCHAFER,
No. 26 South Tennessee Avenue.

PIMPLES REMOVED.

LOS ANGELES, Cal., August 25, 1897.

To T. Foo Yuen:

My daughter was troubled with pimples on her face, and they not only looked badly, but were a constant source of annoyance. Many different remedies were tried without success, and finally she placed herself under the care of Dr. Foo, who treated her by purifying the blood. After about four months the pimples entirely disappeared, and after she had stopped taking medicine the effect was more beneficial. W. G. COGSWELL, 1138 S. Flower street.

The following from Miss Zella Bracewell of Ontario, Cal., explains itself:

ONTARIO, Cal., September, 1896.

T. Foo Yuen, Los Angeles, Cal.

Dear sir: I came to California in the fall of 1893 in hopes that change of climate would improve my health, but it was no avail, and I continued to grow worse. I then began treatment with our local doctors, and was under their care for a year, receiving but very little benefit. I was born with a very poor constitution, and have been troubled with spinal affection from a child, and of late years it has caused me much suffering. I also had nervous prostration, severe headaches, gas on the stomach and other troubles. My blood was very poor and my system greatly poisoned.

Hearing of Dr. Foo, and of some of the cures he had effected, I decided simply out of curiosity, to see him, and was greatly surprised when he placed his finger on my pulse and gave me a correct diagnosis of my case without asking but one question, and that was my age.

From that time I had a great desire to take treatment of him, believing he could help if not cure me. I find his medicines are very searching, cleansing and purifying the blood and invigorating the whole system. I know personally of many who have been cured and greatly benefited by his treatment.

Last September, while under Dr. Foo's treatment, I caught a severe cold and had an attack of tonsilitis, which poisoned my whole system, but through the skill of Dr. Foo I recovered rapidly, and am now well of it. Several friends told me that they did not expect me to live, and some people said the Chinese doctor was killing me, but I have proved to them that he has done the opposite—saved my life. I have gained thirty pounds in weight under his treatment, and am now enjoying better health than I have for years.

I can truly say I believe Dr. Foo has done more for me than any physician that I have any knowledge of could have done, and my gratitude to him is unbounded.   ZELLA BRACEWELL.

The following is of interest in this connection:

REDLANDS, Cal., October 16, 1897.

The Foo and Wing Herb Company:

Gentlemen: My experience with Dr. Foo has probably been one of the most remarkable among his many patients. In 1891 I commenced to have womb trouble, and consulted physicians of both schools in Redlands. They all pronounced it a case of tumor, and their diagnosis was doubtless correct, but their treatment was not as satisfactory; for I tried a great many remedies and prescriptions without beneficial result. The physicians desired to perform an operation, but I dreaded the pain and danger and would not consent. As this seemed to be the last resort within their reach I stopped doctoring entirely and was ill all of the time until 1893, when I heard of Dr. Foo, who had just then come to Redlands. I noticed that people of education and intelligence consulted him, and I heard a great deal about his success in the diseases of women. So I finally decided to go and see him, and to ask him to give me an examination and opinion.

He asked me no questions whatever, but informed me that there was a tumor and congealed blood in the womb. I was very much surprised at the correctness of his diagnosis, which corresponded with all that I knew before of my condition, and I at once decided to take his medicine. I continued it for three months; sometimes I appeared to be a little better, sometimes worse. My family were nearly discouraged at the end of this time, but I saw so many of Dr. Foo's patients who were doing well, but a few of them not progressing very fast, that I decided to keep on. I continued to take the herbs for about eleven months in all. Then I stopped them entirely, and at that time I looked and felt better than I had been for many years. I have found that the great improvement made has been permanent.

Since that time I have taken these remedies at intervals, for colds and other troubles, and have always found them thoroughly satisfactory.   MRS. M. M. REEDER.

A VOICE FROM THE KLONDIKE.

As an illustration of what our remedies accomplish for women we present the following extract from a letter written by Alice Rollins Crane to a friend in Los Angeles:

"DAWSON CITY, Northwest Territory, Oct. 10, 1898.

"Tell Mr. Hazard to say to Dr. T. Foo Yuen that my health has never been better, and that I give him the credit for it. After years of suffering, and that without hope of recovery, he cured me, gave me a new lease of life, so that I could finish my work. My work in Alaska for the Smithsonian Institute, among the tribes of Indians, has called for the most severe exposures and privations. I have now been in this country nearly a year, and for ninety days at a time the thermometer has ranged from zero to 45 deg. below, and I have really enjoyed it. I have often walked eighteen miles one day and returned the second day, without any symptoms of the old trouble, and I have a feeling of gratitude for the doctor. He has brought to our shores a science which was born of centuries of medical evolutions, and which puts the modern 'fake' to shame. I wish he had a branch in Dawson, now we have some 16,000 people and plenty of sickness.

"ALICE ROLLINS CRANE."

A SPLENDID ILLUSTRATION

of the value of the herbal system of medicine is afforded by Mrs. Crane's case. As in thousands of cases, Mrs. Crane's illness was gradual deterioration, growing from bad to worse, for several years. During all that time she was unable to secure any permanent relief, and came at last to a point where she was utterly at a loss. It was evident that something must be done if her life was to be saved, but she had no confidence in the remedies offered her by numerous physicians. She was finally advised by physicians whom she believed to be competent that only a certain very severe and difficult surgical operation would save her life. But, upon careful investigation, she discovered that in this operation there was only one chance in eight for her life. In other words, of every eight women who submit to this operation seven die from its effects. Mrs. Crane further learned that, of those who recover, the average length of life subsequent to the operation is eight years. This was truly a pleasant prospect for a thoroughly sick and discouraged woman to contemplate.

In this crisis of her affairs Mrs. Crane happened to hear of the Foo and Wing Herb Company, and determined to consult them. The pulse diagnosis which she received and the information in reference to the methods employed and the remedies used appealed at once to her sturdy common sense, and she accepted implicitly the statement of the doctors that they could cure her, without risk and danger; and without any operation whatever. That the result was fully up to the promises made is abundantly shown by the letter quoted above. Here is a case that is absolutely beyond dispute. Mrs. Crane's great work among the Apaches and other Indian tribes, her elaborate studies of their histories, traditions and ways of life, and her writings in reference to these are matters familiar to hundreds of people in Los Angeles. Equally well known is her present mission to the frozen North, whither she has gone as a representative of the Smithsonian Institute and of a syndicate of eastern publications. There can be no mistake and no humbug about a case so well attested as is this. All of the testimonials that we print are genuine, but few of them are so tersely written and so unusual as is this letter from Mrs. Crane.

FOR THE SPECIAL BENEFIT OF WOMEN.

The facts in this letter are of interest to every one, but of special interest to women. For they prove, what we have asserted before, that women are not absolutely dependent upon the knife for relief from their peculiar ills. The prevalent craze for surgical operations in treating the diseases of women is a fad pure and simple. It is as unnecessary as it is cruel and ineffective. We have remedies that meet these cases fully. They accomplish by gradual processes of absorption and nutrition what cannot be accomplished by violent and quicker means. Nature does not work in a hurry in the cure of these diseases. They require a little time if a cure is to be safe and sure, and the summary methods of the modern surgeon are as far removed as possible from natural methods.

CHAPTER VIII.

HOW TO CURE A COLD.

ONLY ONE SAFE AND SATISFACTORY METHOD—SIMPLE COLDS THE ORIGIN OF FATAL DISEASES.

DIFFICULTIES IN CURING OR PREVENTING THEM—ATMOSPHERIC INFLUENCES IN CREATING EPIDEMICS OF INFLUENZA—RESULTS OF MISTAKES IN TREATMENT AND DIET—SLIGHT ATTACKS MADE INFINITELY WORSE—THE SAFE AND EFFICIENT SYSTEM OF THE FOO & WING HERB COMPANY—VEGETABLE SPECIFICS BY FAR THE BEST.

Half the diseases that kill people originate in simple colds. Everybody knows by experience what a cold is, for everybody takes cold. A warm and genial climate is not a safeguard. People take cold in California as easily as they do in the East, and a dry winter is more productive of evil in this respect than a winter with a heavier rainfall. In dry years there is a greater contrast between sun and shade, day and night. And people are more careless because they erroneously think they are safer.

In its simplest form a cold is a disease, which runs a regular course and usually terminates in about two weeks. In its more severe results it ends in la grippe, influenza, pneumonia and various forms of fever such as typhoid. Sometimes a cold arises simply from exposure, through a chilling of a portion of the body, a consequent congestion and interruption of the circulation, then comes fever which gives rise to poison in the system. If the patient is strong enough to throw these poisons off there may be no serious permanent injury. If he is weak or predisposed to other diseases the cold marks the beginning of a more severe, often fatal malady. Even the simplest cold is some injury. Even if cured it leaves its mark upon the constitution and makes the next cold easier. After a little there is a decided tendency, which ends in consumption or some other virulent disorder.

DIFFICULTY OF A CURE.

Considering the prevalence of colds and the long experience of physicians in treating them one would suppose that they could be quickly and easily cured. They could be and would be if the medicine could fulfil its promises. But medicine don't do anything of the kind. Everybody who has ever had a cold knows this. If you take it right at the very start perhaps a big dose of quinine or a hot lemonade or some other of the advertised cures may bring relief. But few people are smart enough to take a cold at the start. It is human nature to wait till it develops, hoping in the meantime that it will go away itself. But it never does. When pain begins to be felt, and there is headache, bones ache and fever, then heavy doses of some powerful mineral remedy are usually taken, and that settles the question by making the trouble worse. The powerful drugs causes irritation and greater fever. Then nature has to contend with the cold and the medicine, too. The cold then has to "run its course." It may settle in one part of the body, as in the lungs, and cause intense inflammation. Or it may go all through the body and cause general depression and pains from head to foot. In either case nature requires time to rally her forces and drive the malady from the system. Sometimes nature is too weak and then there is "quick consumption," or some other destructive disease.

PREDISPOSITION TO COLDS.

Many people take cold very easily. They are naturally of delicate constitutions or else they are neglectful of their health. They live too closely within doors, take too little exercise and neglect the care of the skin, which becomes unduly sensitive. Then very little exposure results in a cold. An improper diet is a very common cause. This makes the blood impure, retards the vital processes and clogs the system with impurities which hinder the circulation. The result is a depressed state of vitality and a weakened nervous system. Consequently the person takes a cold easily and gets rid of it with difficulty. Every cold so taken makes the way easier for another, until a slight change in the temperature of a room, a slight exposure to a draught or a trifling wetting brings on the pernicious result. There is only one way to overcome this predisposition. The blood must be purified, the circulation must be quickened, the diet regulated, digestion assisted, the normal action of the skin restored. Then the individual stands a chance of resisting disease.

ATMOSPHERIC INFLUENCES.

Sometimes colds are epidemic. La grippe and influenza travel in the atmosphere. They are contagious, so that when one member of a family is attacked all the others are pretty certain to suffer. There are millions of germs of these diseases floating in the air. Climatic conditions beyond the control of man govern their development. When these diseases are epidemic everybody breathes the germs. The strong may escape without injury, because they cast the germs off at once. But those who are weak, for any reason, or pre-disposed, fail to get rid of the germs. If the person has already been a frequent sufferer from colds, or if he has catarrh or asthma, then the germs find tissues, in the lungs and air passages which are irritated, congested or ulcerated. These surfaces are favorable to their lodgment and development. They find a home and grow by millions. The result is influenza, la grippe, pneumonia, lung fever or some similar disorder. The weaker the person is the harder to dislodge these germs and to prevent their continued development. If his system is already debilitated or impure, he has a hard struggle, which very often ends in a chronic disease or in death.

SIMPLE CASES AGGRAVATED BY IMPROPER TREATMENT.

In thousands of cases, colds, which would be trifling in their results if let alone, or treated in a rational way, are converted into critical disorders by incompetent and improper treatment. Mistakes in diet alone do great harm. Persons suffering from even a slight cold should be extremely careful of their diet. The lighter this is, the better. The portions of the food assimilated into the blood are carried to the lungs before they are taken to the other organs. If they are of a heavy or irritating, or too stimulating character, they create greater irritation where there is already too much. Meat soups, in particular, tend to clog the lungs. Powerful drugs and poisonous remedies of all kinds have a similar effect. They create greater irritation and fever. Whisky and other stimulants, which are very often prescribed, are simply adding fuel to a fire. They cannot lessen the inflammation; they produce more intense inflammation. The action of the skin is impeded, and colds often settle in the kidneys. Hence, with the natural outlets for poisons impeded, it is certainly illogical to add poisons in the way of so-called remedies. Yet this is often the course pursued. And the patient gets worse and worse, while firmly believing that he is doing all in his power to get well.

TRY A MORE RATIONAL REMEDY.

Anyone who reads carefully the above paragraphs—which simply set forth the facts within the knowledge and experience of all—will understand why the Oriental Herbal remedies are more efficient in curing colds and all diseases originating in colds than any others known. The action of these remedies has been so often discussed in the public press that almost everybody understands it now. People know that these specifics are harmless, that they remove poisons from the human body instead of adding more poisons to the poisons already there and already doing a great deal of harm, and that they act favorably and promptly upon all the vital organs. They quicken the circulation and drive the cold back to the skin when it disappears. They assist nature in getting rid of all the poisonous products of the cold and of the resulting inflammation, and, finally, they are nourishing. They keep up the strength and to a great extent, they take the place of food for a time. They are readily assimilated by the stomach, promote the secretion of the gastric juices and assist digestion. They are not irritants which nature must get rid of, but simply agents for cleansing, for renewing and for giving strength.

If a cold is treated at the outset these remedies quickly work a cure. In two or three days the sufferer is as well as ever again. If the cold has become firmly seated, a longer time is required. But nature is helped in such a way that permanent injury is prevented. There is no danger that the cold will settle in a vital organ and produce acute inflammation or a chronic condition that may end in a disease dangerous to life.

TESTIMONIALS.

The following letter is from a former attache of the Los Angeles Health Office, who was threatened with an attack of typhoid fever as a result of taking cold. Mr. Crane says:

S. P. Bagg, Pres.; A. R. Crane, Sec.; L. P. Crane, Mgr.
BLUE BOOK PUBLISHING COMPANY,
    Of California.
  Office: 242 Wilcox Block.

LOS ANGELES, Cal., Sept. 7, 1897.

The Foo and Wing Herb Company, Los Angeles, Cal.: Feeling grateful for services rendered me in case of serious sickness, I beg to add to the long list of cures you have made through your method of treatment. I was, as you know, in the incipient stages of typhoid fever, having been unable to attend to my business for several weeks. Your treatment in ten days entirely removed the fever and brought my whole body into a normal state, full of vigor and ambition.

I am convinced you have a method of treatment which is effective and which leaves no bad effects through the system. Science seems to have almost entirely obliterated the old methods of practice, and is giving way to the herb, with which, I believe, the Almighty intended to heal the countless millions of suffering humanity. I congratulate you upon your success, and honor the ancient school of China, with its thousand years of ripe experience. Truth is all powerful and the scoffer cannot down it. Very truly yours,

L. P. CRANE,
Ex-Deputy Health Officer, Los Angeles, Cal.

STATEMENT OF A REMARKABLE CASE.

LOS ANGELES, California, October 21, 1897.

The Foo and Wing Herb Company, Los Angeles—Gentlemen: On the 15th day of last July I was taken sick with an illness which finally became very severe, as I was unable to leave my bed for nine weeks. I had doctored with Dr. Foo on a former occasion, but, not understanding the serious condition that might develop from the beginning of the present illness, I did not send for him at first, but consulted an American doctor. I had at this time a great deal of pain, but no fever or other alarming symptoms. The physician whom I called was unable to determine exactly what the trouble was. He said that it was very obscure, but he thought that it was a gall-stone in the gall bladder. He prescribed for me, and I took his remedies for five days, during which time I rapidly grew worse.

Finding that I was getting no better, and this doctor having done for me everything that seemed to be in his power, I consulted another doctor, who at first thought I had typhoid fever, but afterward concluded that it was a case of appendicitis. I do not know what he treated me for, but I do know that he gave me medicines which I took. This lasted for about ten days longer, when the physician frankly informed me that he really did not know what the trouble was, and desired to consult with another doctor. But my husband and friends did not think that this was worth while. I then sent for Dr. Foo, who came to see me. At this time my husband and friends had entirely given me up, and did not think that I could live for twenty-four hours. When he saw me, Dr Foo also thought that the case had reached a point where it had become very serious, and that all he could do was to relieve the pain for a few days at the most. However, he gave me some herb teas, which I commenced to take and began to improve from the very first dose. It was nearly six weeks, however, before I was able to leave my bed, as I had become very much reduced in strength before Dr. Foo prescribed for me.

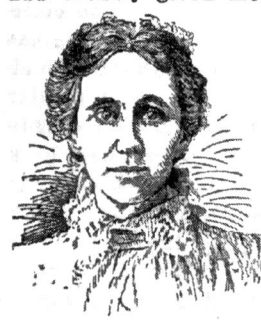

MRS. PORTMAN.

I have been taking treatment of Dr. Foo

ever since; have completely regained my health and look and feel as well as ever in my life.

Both I myself and all of my friends believe that I would not be alive today if I had not consulted Dr. Foo and received help from his remedies.

Dr. Foo said that the case was simply a slight attack of malaria and could easily have been cured had the proper remedies been given at the start.
MRS. P. N. PORTMAN,
231 North Anderson street.

As Mrs. Portman's nurse during the illness above mentioned and described, I know that all the particulars herein given are true, without exaggeration, as therein stated. MRS. E. M. BELL.

We, the undersigned, neighbors and friends of Mrs. P. N. Portman, were acquainted with the circumstances of her recent severe illness and hereby certify to the truth of the above statement of those circumstances.

LOTTIE BAHRES, 209 North Anderson street,
MRS C. SEARS, 229 North Anderson street, city.

The following letter is from Mrs. A. A. Mayhew, a lady who has had a great deal of experience with this system of medicine. She says:

The Foo and Wing Herb Company: Gentlemen—It is with pleasure that I testify to the prompt and speedy cure effected by the use of your herbs. I have been subject to a bronchial cough from childhood, which of late years has confined me to the house the greater part of the winter season. And now, at the age of 78, to find a medicine which will in the winter season, even when accompanied by a severe attack of la grippe, entirely relieve such a cough and leave the system in a vigorous condition, is a great satisfaction.

Respectfully,

MRS. A. A. MAYHEW.

No. 4 Barnard Park, Los Angeles, Cal., January 31, 1897.

John Motherspaw of San Bernardino writes:

SAN BERNARDINO, Cal., May 15, 1897.

The Foo and Wing Herb Company, Los Angeles: Gentlemen—My only experience with Dr. Foo's method of treatment was very satisfactory indeed, as it cured me of a very severe attack of la grippe, when everything else that I had tried had failed. This was in January of this year. La grippe was epidemic in this part of the country and many people were dying from it and from pneumonia, which was what it went to in many cases.

After I was taken ill I tried several remedies, but kept getting worse, and this continued for two or three weeks. Everybody knows what this disease is, so that I need not try to tell how much I suffered from it. I was seriously alarmed at my condition, and when Dr. Foo's remedies were called to my attention I concluded to try them as a last resort. They helped me at once, and I gradually became better until, in about a month, I was entirely well. They not only cured the la grippe, but they seemed to help me in other ways, so that, at the end of the course of treatment, I was feeling better than I had felt for ten years before. JOHN MOTHERSPAW.

Following is an additional testimonial on this subject:

REDLANDS, California, October 4, 1897.

The Foo and Wing Herb Company, Los Angeles: Gentlemen—My experience with Dr. Foo as a physician has been very satisfactory. About two years ago this coming December I took a very hard cold, which settled on my lungs and developed into a troublesome cough. I tried various remedies without receiving any benefit. After a little I went to Dr. Foo and took about two months' treatment. In that time my cough was cured and my lungs since then have been stronger than ever. I have known of many other patients who have been cured by Dr. Foo's remedies.

I have read Dr. Foo's different publications, and I know that he is the first man who has ever explained the Chinese System of Medicine for the benefit of the American people. I believe that, in these publications, he is accomplishing a great deal of good.

F. A. M'CRARY.

The following is brief, but to the point:

CHICAGO, Ill., May 16, 1897.

This is to certify that I appreciate with heartfelt thanks the great improvement after taking treatment from T. Foo Yuen for the disease of bronchitis and la grippe, of which I am entirely relieved. Advising others to give him a trial which I think will prove beneficial in all cases, I will gratefully remain, Yours truly,

MRS. JENNIE SIMPSON,
446 Medill avenue, Chicago, Ill.

Another letter of similar import:

LOS ANGELES, Cal., May 12, 1897.

After a severe attack of la grippe, which left me feeling miserable, I am taking Dr. Foo's medicine, which is greatly benefiting me.

Yours truly, MRS. A. M. CARY, Magnolia avenue.

AN ATTACK OF PNEUMONIA CURED.

TEHACHAPI, Kern County, Cal., Oct. 28, 1901.

The Foo and Wing Herb Company, Los Angeles, Cal.:

Gentlemen—Your cure of my daughter of an attack of pneumonia last summer is a splendid illustration of what your remedies can accomplish in acute diseases. The child is now about seven years of age. She took a severe cold which developed into a very high fever, rapid pulse, extreme weakness and all the symptoms of pneumonia.

Although living at Tehachapi, some distance from Los Angeles, we knew of your methods of treatment and at once decided to bring the little girl to you. This was done at once. You stated that you would try your best remedies and thought that you could "grow up the natural juices of the body" and overcome the fever, which seemed to be burning up the lungs. Your remedies accomplished this in about a week, when the child was able to sit up, and in another week she had regained much of her strength. We continued the treatment for about six weeks, when she seemed to be perfectly well, and has remained so since.

This cure of a disorder which is usually very quickly fatal has shown us that your remedies are just as effective in acute cases as in those that are chronic, and has strengthened the confidence which we already had in the great merits of your herbal remedies.

ELLERT M. LOOMIS.

The child above referred to is my granddaughter. I am familiar with the facts stated and know that they are true.

C. A. LOOMIS,
1430 Arapahoe street, Los Angeles.

CONVINCED OF THE MERITS OF THE SYSTEM.

SAN BERNARDINO, California, October 28, 1901.

This is to certify that I was cured of a severe cold in one week's time by Dr. Tom Leong of the Foo and Wing Herb Company. I consider the Chinese herbs superior to all other remedies, both for acute and chronic diseases, and I recommend them to all sufferers.

I have seen the effects of this system of medicine in a great many cases, having known a number of the patrons of the Foo and Wing Herb Company, some of whom were afflicted with very severe and dangerous ailments which had been pronounced incurable by many physicians. The number of cures that I have seen, about which there can be no question whatever, has fully convinced me of the great merit of this system of healing by purely vegetable remedies.

W. E. BOTTOMS.

CURED OF CHRONIC SORE THROAT.

LOS ANGELES, Cal., Nov. 26, 1901.

To Whom This May Concern:

I have been suffering with sore throat for over twelve years and have been treated by a great many doctors, but none could cure me, and all have told me they could only relieve me. Not until I consulted Tom Leong of the Foo and Wing Herb Company could I get any permanent benefit. After taking their herbal remedies for three weeks I was entirely cured. And I have not felt any more symptoms of the sore throat since.

This treatment has also done me a great deal of good in other ways, and I can highly recommend it to any person afflicted with any disease.   MRS. L. BACH.

We know the above to be correct in every respect.

J. BACH,
MRS. WM. W. PADRICK.

FOUND THE TREATMENT BENEFICIAL.

LOS ANGELES, Cal., Oct. 12, 1901.

This is to certify that I appreciate with heartfelt thanks the great improvement after taking three months treatment from Dr. T. Foo Yuen for the headache, from which I had suffered for twenty years, and had tried many physicians and they had done me no good; and a year ago I took a heavy cold that settled on my lungs and developed into a troublesome cough. I could not sleep at night, and now I am entirely relieved, and would advise others to give him a trial, which I think will prove beneficial in all cases. I gratefully remain,

Yours truly,   ALICE PICO, 1538 Kerney St.

A WORD OF APPRECIATION.

LOS ANGELES, Cal. Oct. 26, 1901.

This is to certify that I have known Dr. Tom Leong, vice-president of the Foo and Wing Herb Company for the past year and a half. Myself and others who are acquainted with Dr. Tom Leong consider him a physician of unusual ability, well versed in the herbal system of medication and in diagnosis by the pulse, and a valuable member of the corporation of which he is vice-president. Although he has not yet been as long in this country as his brother, Dr. T. Foo Yuen, yet he is already establishing an excellent reputation for the treatment of the diseases of the American people.

GEORGE MILLER,
2112 Enterprise street, Los Angeles, Cal.

CURED OF STOMACH TROUBLE.

DETROIT, Mich.,
December 31, 1901.

THE FOO AND WING HERB CO., LOS ANGELES:

Gentlemen—I was suffering with stomach trouble and general debility; was very much run down and weighed only 77 pounds, when 17 years of age. I was treated by Drs. T. Foo Yuen and Tom Leong for three months and my appetite and strength returned and my weight increased to 125 pounds, and have been well ever since and now weigh 150 pounds. My eyes were too weak for use, but are in good condition now and am attending school and working hard, and my old complaints have entirely left me, and am stronger than ever before in my life. I shall always be very grateful to you for the benefits of your treatment and gladly recommend it to any who are suffering as I was. There is certainly something in your herbal remedies more effective than the mixtures of our American doctors, whom I have tried without any success.

Yours very sincerely,,
GEO. B. DANA.

1026 Fourth avenue.

MALARIAL POISONING.

The Origin of Many Diseases—Microbes that Play Havoc with the Human Body—Views of a Prominent Physician of New York City—A Discussion Thereof by a Member of the Foo & Wing Herb Company—How the Oriental System Cures Malaria—The Effects of Climatic Influences on Growing Old Early—Californians at a Disadvantage—Illustrative Cases.

People have very hazy notions about malaria. There are so many symptoms of disease that doctors ascribe to malaria that the mind of the average citizen gets confused. The common understanding is that malaria is a poison produced by dampness or filth, which finds its way into the human system and makes trouble. So far as it goes, this understanding of malaria is correct. But it does not tell the whole truth.

The New York Journal in a recent issue wrote up the subject of malaria in connection with certain improvements that were being made in New York, during the progress of which miles of streets in the most fashionable portion of the city were torn up. The Journal contended that this wholesale tearing up of streets would inevitably give rise to an epidemic of malaria. It quoted, in support of this contention, the celebrated physician, Dr. Cyrus Edson, and took numerous samples of earth from the excavations to chemists, who analyzed them and reported that they were full of the germs of disease. Illustrations were printed of these germs, enlarged many times, showing the terrible little monsters which enter the blood and play havoc there. Dr. Edson said: "Malaria is the one ailment that opens the gateway of the system to disease and possible death. The germ of malaria has never yet been found outside the human body, but physicians have learned that it always makes its appearance when such a state of affairs exists as is caused by a condition of the streets like that of Fifth avenue and in other sections of New York." Among the diseases that follow malaria are la grippe, typhoid fever, consumption, pneumonia, diphtheria and cholera infantum.

THE ORIENTAL VIEW.

Mr. George W. Hazard, a gentleman who was much interested in this subject, and is also familiar with the Oriental System of Medicine and the opinions of Oriental physicians in general, took a copy of the Journal to one of the members of the Foo and Wing Herb Company, and asked his opinion on Dr. Edson's views. Knowing that the most ancient system of medical practice extant among men is usually found to be in harmony with the most advanced and modern ideas upon theoretical points, although differing radically in the use of remedial agents, Mr. Hazard was curious to know whether this fact would hold good in the present instance. The Oriental physician emphatically endorsed the opinion of the great New York physician, and stated that he himself had studied the bacilli of malaria through the use of the microscope. "Malaria injures the people in many different ways, and causes many different forms of sickness," he said.

THREE FORMS OF MALARIAL POISONING.

"In a general way," said Dr. Li Wing, "there are three stages of malarial poisoning. It may settle in the skin, in the flesh, or in the nerves and muscles. The poison is easily removed from the skin; is harder to remove from the flesh, and is hardest of all to remove when it settles in the nerves and inner tissues of the muscles. From these it frequently attacks the vital organs, and then there is great difficulty in accomplishing a cure."

THE PROPER REMEDIES.

"Dr. Edson," Mr. Hazard remarked, "makes no mention of a means of cure. He describes the poison and tells what it will do, but he does not tell how to get rid of it. What are your ideas on that subject?"

"I think," was the reply, "that most doctors treat malarial troubles with quinine. In some cases there may be relief from quinine. In others there is none. Remedies are needed which will drive the poison out of the blood and the nerves and tissues, and send it back to the skin, and then it will disappear. But quinine does not have this expansive power. It acts just the opposite way. It tends to bring everything inward, to contract. The vitality of the patient must also be aroused, so that his natural powers of resistance to the disease will work in harmony with the remedies given. The best remedies for this purpose are the herbal remedies, because they assist all the vital organs and work the poison out of the body."

CHILLS AND FEVER.

"Why do people suffering from the ague first have a chill and then have fever?" Mr. Hazard inquired.

"This is a conflict between the vitality of the patient and the poison of malaria. When the poison is the stronger there is a chill and depression of the vital forces. Their action is so far hindered that the body cannot keep itself warm. When nature arouses all her strength to expel the poison, inflammation or fever is caused. In this condition the natural power is the heat which goes through all the nerves, the muscles and the pores of the body. When the poison wins there are chills; when the natural power wins, there is fever. If the fever comes first and is followed by a chill, that shows that there is not strength or vitality enough to fight against the poison, and that the poison is getting too strong a hold upon the body. These cases are very difficult to cure. We treated many cases of this sort in San Francisco, many of whom came from Florida, from Boston, New York, Chicago and other large eastern cities. The climate of the east is more severe than that of California, and the forms of malaria resulting therefrom are also more severe."

MALARIA AND CLIMATE.

"How does the climate of California differ from that of other states?" asked Mr. Hazard.

"The weather of California is clearer and softer," was the reply. "The malaria originating here is less destructive and there is less of the ague form. Still there is some. The cold nights of our summers keep the malarial poison in check. If it were not for these there would be much more of this sort of sickness, because heat gives rise to malaria as well as dampness. The climate of California has many advantages, but it has some disadvantges. In one day, even in this State, there are many changes which come quickly, and there is a great difference between the temperatures of the morning and the night and between day and night, and these sudden changes cause people to take cold very easily. The dryness in the atmosphere affects the skin, and the dry south wind which blows so much of the time affects the oil in the skin of the face.

ON GROWING OLD EARLY.

"The people of this State look old sooner than they do in the East. There is eight or nine years' difference in the appearance of the ladies as between California and the East, and the difference is in favor of the Eastern ladies. People in the East who are 40 years old look younger than those of 30 in California. This is largely because of climatic conditions, a result of the dryness of the atmosphere. This is also largely influenced by diet. The people of California do not care for boiled and steamed meats, which keep the natural juices of the body good and control the natural heat. They eat too much roast and fried meat. For this reason there is too much heat in the system and this also causes the people to look old early.

"If the people of California would use steamed meats, rice and similar foods they would help the gastric juices and keep the skin soft all of the time. Then they would not look old so early in life. This is the way the Chinese in San Francisco retain their youthful appearance. None of them look old early except those who are addicted to opium. Their diet is wholesome and when they are a little ill and are required to take medicines, instead of taking stimulants and concentrated substances which create fever in the human body, they use vegetable remedies which promote the flow of natural juices and assist the action of the vital organs. This keeps the skin smooth and soft and full of natural oils. The wrinkles of age and ill health are prevented. The man continues young. The whole secret is in a healthful diet and a harmless system of medication.

TYPICAL CASES OF MALARIA.

"The same reasoning applies to many diseases, and especially to malaria. If the body is kept in a healthful condition by proper food it will resist the attacks of the microbes which cause the malarial poisoning. And if this disease has once become seated, remedies must be given which will cleanse the system and make it normal. Take the case of John Myers of this city. His sickness commenced from malaria. He had chills and fever. Afterward the poison settled in the bowels and from these went to the feet so that he could not walk; but after it had gone to his feet he had no more chills and fever; still it was the same poison. Our treatment and remedies cleansed the poison out of his system and removed it entirely through the skin, and also caused the natural juices to grow and to control the inflammation. After two months' treatment he commenced to walk, and was soon able to walk half a block without his crutches, for the first time in two years. This showed that the poison had been compelled to release its hold upon the nerves and muscles, thus permitting them to do their work again.

"James Campbell lives at San Bernardino, in a hot climate. Nevertheless he contracted malaria through working among the trees and fruits. After irrigation or a rain or a fog the heat of the sun caused rapid evaporation of the moisture in the earth and produced malaria in the atmosphere. Mr. Campbell was ill for ten years, at first with chills and fever, afterwards with rheumatism. Quinine and similar remedies checked the chills, but did not remove the poison, and he was never well until after a course of our remedies had expelled the poison from his system.

"Thomas Stewart of Redlands contracted malaria from improper diet. Too much fried and roast meats created inflammation which caused an excessive desire for raw fruits and cold water. These caused a chill and dampness in the system which joined with the existing inflammation in making trouble. He first seemed to have a cold and then a fever. Then the poison went to his feet and caused them to swell. He could not bear the weight of a fly upon them or the jarring of a person walking past his bed. He took a great deal of medicine, which only made him worse, and he came very near dying. Our herb teas cured him. We treated him only for malaria, although, in his case, the trouble did not arise from changes in the weather or climate. By using the microscope we find in such cases the same conditions in the blood, saliva and other secretions as in cases of malaria from climatic changes. The pulse is also the same. In either case the accumulations of poison in the system must be removed before there can be any improvement."

The following letters illustrate the points brought out in the above article. The first one shows a cure of

A REMARKABLE CASE OF PARALYSIS.

1412 North Main street, Los Angeles, Cal., October 18, 1897.
The Foo and Wing Herb Company, Los Angeles:

Gentlemen—Two years and four months ago I was taken with an

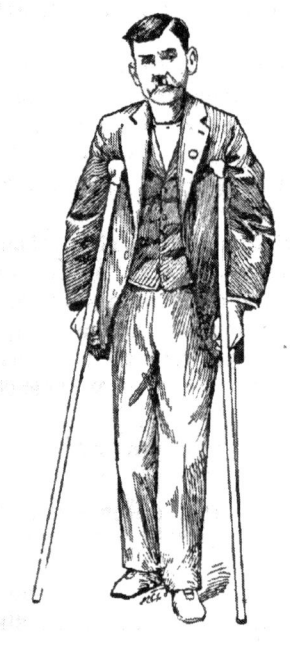
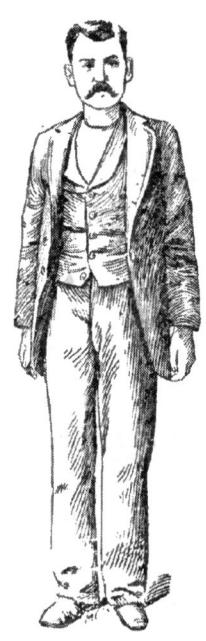

attack of la grippe, which was followed by chills and fever. The fever kept on for months. During the first three weeks I had two physicians, who did what they could do for me, but with so little effect that I completely lost the use of my limbs, at the end of three weeks, and was confined to my bed. I could not help myself at all and was fed by others. For two months I was not expected to live.

At the end of the first month I secured a new physician who prescribed principally morphine and strychnine. I took a solution of the latter drug in quantities amounting to ninety drops a day, and three doses of morphine every night, a grain and a half at a does, which was required to give me any rest at all. In all I had eleven different physicians, and also spent ten days at the county hospital, but while there I took no medicine worth mentioning, although I had good care and nursing.

I finally recovered far enough to leave my bed, but went on crutches, which I have been compelled to use for about two years. May 25th of the present year I went to the hot springs at San Juan Capistrano. I remained there for three months and took the hot sulphur baths. I received some benefit from this treatment, but was not cured.

Seven weeks ago I commenced your treatment and have received more benefit in this period of seven weeks than in all of the previous doctoring and hot springs treatment. I can now walk about half a block without my crutches, and am better in every way. I have gained in both strength and weight, and my appetite is now good, for the first time since I was first taken sick.

My different doctors called my trouble muscular rehumatism, paralysis, nervous debility and various other things. Your physicians considered it a slight stroke of paralysis, and their diagnosis has certainly been shown to be correct by the results of their prescriptions. All of my friends are astonished at the progress that I have made in the past few weeks.   JOHN MYERS.

COMPLICATIONS RESULTING FROM MALARIA.

REDLANDS, Cal., October 4, 1897.

The Foo and Wing Herb Company, Los Angeles:

Gentlemen—I feel that my long acquaintance with Dr. Foo justifies me in speaking very positively of his success in curing disease.

I first became acquainted with him something over two years ago, when I consulted him through the advice of friends in Redlands who had been cured by him of different diseases, and knew what he could do. I had then been sick for ten years and had given up all hopes of ever recovering, or of receiving help from physicians or from medicines. Dr. Foo diagnosed my case as an accumulation of poisons in the system which involved the stomach, bowels, liver and spleen, the last mentioned organ being very badly affected. These troubles were complicated by catarrh of twenty-six years' standing. I had often been treated for this difficulty, but had never received any benefit.

After talking with Dr. Foo I commenced to take his remedies, and continued them for seven months. When I commenced I was so weak that I could not even unlace my own shoes, and could do no work whatever. In seven weeks from the commencement of my treatment I was able to work. I kept on getting stronger and better, was entirely cured at the end of the seven months, and have been at work ever since upon my ranch. I am satisfied that I would not have found any help for my troubles if I had not consulted Dr. Foo.

JAMES CAMPBELL.

A NEWSPAPER MAN GIVES HIS OPINION.

The following letter is from a gentleman who has seen a great deal of the world on both sides of the water, and was formerly in active business life in London as a writer for and publisher of newspapers. He has now become a permanent resident of Southern California, and lives at present in Riverside. Mr. Wilson says:

261 East Tenth street, Riverside, Cal., Sept. 4, 1896.

Dear Sir: I beg to add my mite of testimony to that of others who have derived benefit from Dr. Foo's treatment. I had been suffering from the ill effects of malarial poisoning for some time, and was persuaded by people who had been cured under the herbal treatment to give Dr. Foo a trial, which I did. I am still taking the medicine, and have derived considerable benefit during the short time I have been under the doctor's care. I have gained fifteen pounds in weight during the two months I have taken the treatment.

Yours truly, A. WILSON.

188   FOO & WING HERB COMPANY

ANOTHER CASE OF PARALYSIS CURED.

The following letter explains itself. It is a convincing proof of what the herbal remedies can accomplish in extreme cases:

SANTA PAULA, Cal., July 18, 1899.

To Whom it May Concern:

This is to certify that I was a sufferer from paralysis from

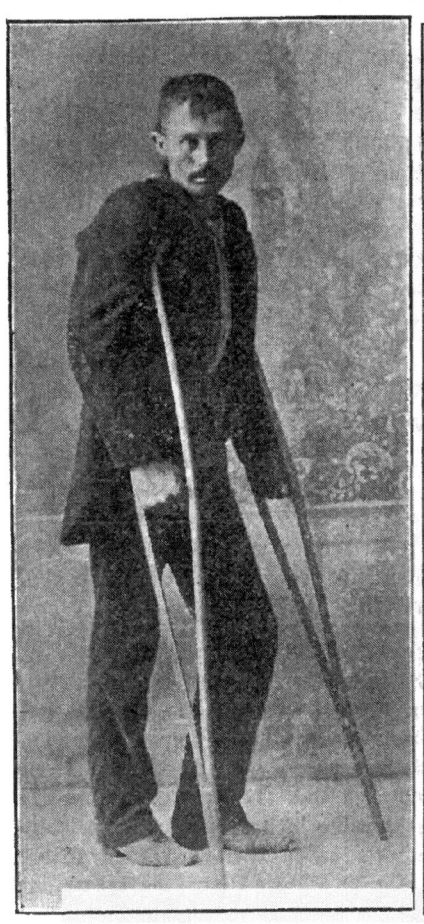
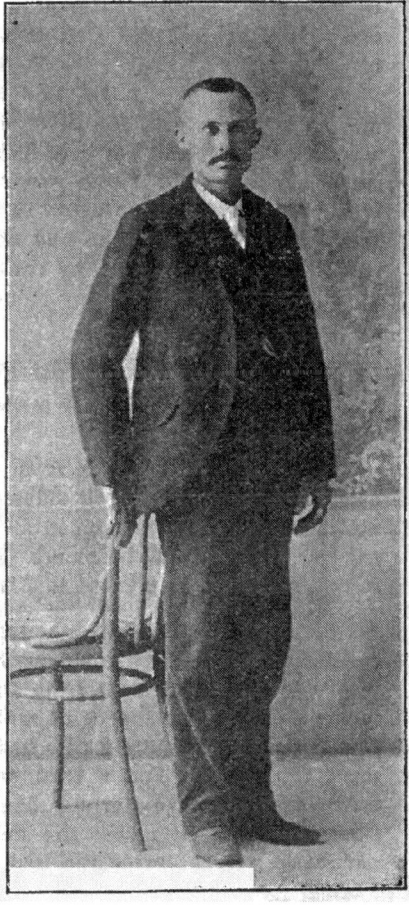

November, 1897, to September, 1898. I tried all sorts of appliances and external remedies, such as electricity, and also consulted the best doctors in San Francisco and Fresno, California, and in New Orleans, La. None of these did me any good, and I gave up all hopes of ever walking again, and did not expect to live long. In September, 1898, I heard of the Foo and Wing Herb Company, and also read the book published by this company which impressed me very much. I was impressed by what was said of the purely herbal treatment, as I had taken no medicines up to this time except strychnine and arsenic, which had poisoned my system almost beyond help.

Dr. Foo gave me a pulse diagnosis and described my condition, but would not promise to cure me. But I commenced the treatment and can now say that, under God, I owe an almost complete recovery to this herbal treatment under the direction of Dr. T. Foo Yuen. I am confident of a permanent and lasting cure in the end. I make this statement in the hope that others suffering as I have suffered will grasp the opportunity to try what I believe to be the only true medicines, pure, healing roots and herbs.   W. T. DENISON.

We, the undersigned, know the above statement to be true in every respect.

W. J. Dechman, P. B. Fulton, C. W. Park, S. D. Cochran and Mrs. H. A. Barr, all of Dinuba, California.

CHAPTER IX.

THE CAUSES AND CURE OF ASTHMA.

There are many things which will produce asthma, and the subject is too large to discuss in full within the compass of a brief chapter.

The first cause of asthma is living in a low, wet place. The air about such places is damp and causes malaria, which goes through the atmosphere. Then the air becomes heavy and too damp, and this being taken into the lungs, remains in them in a heavy, dark vapor, like fog. People who are born in such damp districts do not feel the same bad effects as those who move into them from other sections, because they have become accustomed to breathing this damp air and it does not hurt them so much. It is natural for them, and does not hurt their systems at all. If a person of a strong constitution goes to live in such a place, for the first few months he will feel a little bit weak in the lungs. But after the first few months the system becomes adapted to the weather and the lungs become as strong again as before. The damp air disappears, and there is no sickness. But one whose lungs are naturally weak cannot take care of the damp air. At first the damp air in the lungs is lighter, looks like a fog, then it condenses and becomes congealed and irritates the lungs, forming phlegm. There is a discharge from the nostrils as in catarrh, and, if it continues for some time, the lungs become weaker and the person takes cold easily.

When a person in this condition takes cold there is at once inflammation in the lungs, which dries up the phlegm in the cells of the lungs. This congeals harder than ever, like a little round nut. It looks exactly like a young bee in the honey comb. It stops up the cells of the lungs, and a case of asthma is the result.

A second cause of asthma is taking cold in any way which causes inflammation in the lungs and a cough, if the doctors do not understand how to throw it off and remove it through the skin. If they simply use a strong medicine to relieve the cold, and the inflammation from the cold goes into the lungs and poison from the medicine settles there also, then there is a double trouble, which takes a strong hold upon the lungs and produces asthma. Many cases of this sort have come to our company and have been cured. Some people who come to us say, "I have had pneumonia, which makes my asthma worse," and others say, "I had la grippe ten years ago, and since then I have had asthma," and some say that they have taken a very bad cold, and have had a fever, which caused asthma; some say that they have had asthma since they had an attack of malarial fever. All of these cases show that poisonous remedies were used to cure the cold or other disease; that these poisoned medicines were left in the system and that they caused the asthma.

Third, cases of asthma arise from eating too much fried and roasted meat, and constantly eating food that is too strong and too greasy. From this cause inflammation comes, and this inflammation causes an excessive desire for drinks and for raw fruits. In this way too much cold air is taken into the system, and this dampness and the inflammation work together in causing trouble. Then the stomach produces phlegm and there is heartburn. Then the phlegm from the stomach becomes very thick. It goes through the diaphragm and settles in the lungs, and so produces asthma.

Fourth, some people contract asthma as a result of venereal poisoning. They take mineral remedies to cure this, such as mercury, etc. This goes through the lungs, near the spine, and causes asthma.

Fifth, some people take an ordinary cold, which causes a cough to go through the lungs. The patients do not pay sufficient attention to abstain from eating and drinking, and take too much greasy food, and soups made from strong meats. They feel a little thirsty and they eat an excessive amount of meat soups, partly to relieve the thirst. This food is too strong under the circumstances, and affects the lungs easily. It goes through the lungs more quickly and penetrates deeper than anything else. It closes up the pores of the lungs, and, little by little, gives rise to asthma. Every day, also, the spleen extracts juices from the stomach, which are sent to the lungs by the power of the spleen, but if the pores of the lungs are closed they cannot take up these juices, which become phlegm; then there is a cough, and the asthma becomes worse. If the person's constitution is strong, as in some people, and nature has a little time to help the system, then all the sound pores of the lungs are opened again and become clear, and the cough will stop; but if it has settled near the windpipe the phlegm congeals so hard and the pores are shut up so tightly that there then arises a case of light asthma. But still it is not so severe as to endanger life. But if the constitution is weak and does not respond to the help of nature, then the pores of the lungs are closed and cannot open again; then the lungs have no juices to wet the lower parts, then the liver and kidneys become dry and burn the lungs out, little by little, and the lungs grow smaller and drier all the time. This brings on asthma and sometimes consumption, which is often incurable.

But, if sickness of this sort, in its early stages, is treated by the herbal remedies, to throw off the cold and clear out the phlegm; and if the patient is also very careful about his eating and drinking, lets meat and meat soups and other strong foods alone, even if he feels very weak for a little while, then the cough will be free, the phlegm will be clean and the pores of the lungs will be clear, and there will be no case of asthma. If meats are taken at all during such illness, they should be eaten dry, and soups should be avoided. Then the pores of the lungs will not be locked up so deeply. But even light soups lock up the pores of the lungs very quickly and very tight. This is a good point for every body to understand and remember.

Sixth, a tendency to asthma is frequently inherited from the parents. There is no hardened phlegm as in some of these other cases, but there is what we may call a phlegm poison in the lungs which comes from the father or the mother, and settles in the windpipe, a part of the lungs being covered with it, like a stone covered with moss. The poison looks like the moss on a stone. And there are plenty of spots like this through the lungs. If the constitution of the person is weak, there will be a great many of these spots, and they will keep growing bigger all the time until they take possession of the lungs, which lose their functions. In these cases the child usually dies young. In others, where there is a strong constitution, or even a nature that is of medium strength, if, while the patient is still young, he takes our herbal remedies every time he has an attack of the asthma, taking herb teas and pills alternately, then he will get better. If he takes the medicine for a month or two to get rid of poison, and, when the trouble comes again, takes another course the same as before and gets better again, and so continues, taking a little course of medicine at each attack, after a time the poison will keep getting less and less, and the spots throughout the lungs will keep growing smaller until the child reaches the age of maturity. At this time his whole body grows very fast, and the poison, if his system is pure and in good order, will all disappear. He will never have asthma again all his life. Li Po Tai, in San Francisco, cured a great many cases of this sort.

A TYPICAL CASE OF ASTHMA CURED.

LOS ANGELES, Cal. October 21, 1897.

The Foo and Wing Herb Company, Los Angeles.

Gentlemen: I have been greatly troubled with asthma for the past ten months. Previous to this I had been at work unloading coal from box cars for about three years. The dust from the freight hurt me, and I also frequently took cold from sweating at my work, and then cooling too quickly. I had some difficulty with my lungs for two or three years. Finally it developed into a case of confirmed asthma.

For nine months I could not lie down at all, but slept sitting in a rocking chair. I was entirely exhausted and could not walk half a block. I lost nearly a year's work through sickness. I tried different doctors for about a year before going to Dr. Foo, but had no relief whatever.

About two months ago I consulted Dr. Foo. I then weighed only 118 pounds. I commenced to gain in about a week after beginning the treatment. In two or three weeks I could lie down to sleep. In two weeks I went back to my former work for the Diamond Coal Company. I can now do as good a day's work as ever, feel as strong as ever, and weigh 132 pounds. My health has improved in every way.

My residence is at No. 227 N. Anderson, and is next to that of Mrs. P. W. Portman. I heard of her recent very severe illness. I knew that her doctors gave her up, and that all of her family and friends expected that she would die within a few days. Dr. Foo cured her in a few week's treatment. I knew of this case and decided that the herbal treatment was the proper thing for me if it could accomplish such wonders as that. The result in my own case is a surprise to all of my friends and acquaintances, many of whom thought I would not live very long. Very truly yours,

J. N. SEARS.

A CASE SIMILAR TO THE ABOVE.

LOS ANGELES, Cal., August 28, 1897.

To Whom it May Concern:

I take pleasure in giving a voluntary statement of my experience with Dr. T. Foo Yuen's skill in the treatment of disease. I was taken severely ill last fall, as I thought from taking cold, but the exact nature of the difficulty I did not understand. I could not sleep on account of great distressing in breathing. I also had serious bronchial difficulty and pains in the breast and shoulders. I consulted several physicians of Los Angeles, who pronounced the case consumption, and advised me to go to Arizona, or Old Mexico at once.

As I had already had some experience with the Chinese system of medicine with the celebrated doctor, Li Po Tai, I determined to try it again before going to another state or county, and went to see Dr. T. Foo'Yuen, of whom I had heard very favorable reports. After a careful diagnosis Dr. Foo informed me that my case was one of bad blood poisoning, and not of consumption. The blood rushed to the lungs and caused asthma. I commenced his treatment, and in a very few days the dreadful spasmodic breathing which had prevented me from sleeping, disappeared entirely. In two weeks I discontinued the treatment, and have never had a touch of the trouble since. This may seem incredible to some, but I state the exact truth, and many of my friends are familiar with the circumstances and can testify to my complete cure.

MRS. HELEN W. COE, 316 W. Seventh street.

A PERMANENT CURE OF A DIFFICULT CASE.

We ask the careful reading of the following letter, particularly because it shows that the benefits to be derived from our treatment are permanent and result in a lasting cure and general strengthening of the body:

REDLANDS, Cal., Sept. 5, 1896.

To Whom it May Concern;

January 1, 1895, I gave a testimonal to Dr. Foo in reference to his very successful treatment of my case. I am now ready, some twenty months afterwards, to repeat what I said at that time and to confirm the very favorable report that I then made of Dr. Foo's remarkable skill. My case was somewhat peculiar. I had been troubled for years with asthma. I had spent hundreds of dollars in different places, east and west, with different doctors whose treatment hardly gave even temporary relief and no permanent benefit whatever. I kept growing worse until I was so weak that I could not even get out of my buggy without help.

About this time, May, 1893, I heard of Dr. Foo's skill. I was told about his pulse examinations, and thought that I would try him as a last resort. He examined my pulse and gave me a test treatment and then told me that I could be cured. I continued the treatment for six weeks, and at the end of that time, through the temporary effects of the medicines, I felt worse than when I commenced, and stopped the medicines. I also told a great many people that Dr. Foo was a quack and a humbug.

After a few days, however, I began to feel the good effects of the medicines, and I soon saw that I had made a great mistake in stopping the treatment, as it was the first thing which had done me any good. I asked the doctor to treat me again. He was at first reluctant to do so, but finally consented, and gave me treatment for eight weeks more. At the end of that time I was a new man. My strength gradually returned. I can now handle the sledge hammer as I did in my younger days. I continued to grow stronger for some time and have felt better since my recovery than before I was sick. JOHN M'INTOSH.

LETTER FROM MRS. STRONG.

The Foo, Wing Herb Co.:

Gentlemen: The first I knew about Dr. Foo's skill was in a case of diphtheria. A young girl in my house had this disease, and I was much alarmed for fear my family would take it. Dr. Foo said that he would give me medicine that would prevent it. He did so; none of us took the disease, although I had a very sore throat when I went to him. His medicines cured it so quickly that it seemed wonderful. I then began taking the herbal treatment. I had had bronchitis for over twenty years, and asthma for a longer period, but the doctor's medicines have cured me of both these diseases. I also had chronic rheumatism; in fact, almost all the diseases arising from poisoned blood; but whenever I went to Dr. Foo he had the remedies on hand, and they never failed to do the work promptly and well. I have taken medicine from a great many physicians, but Dr. Foo is the only one whose medicines never failed, and I do not remember of the medicines ever failing in a single instance to accomplish the work for which they were given.

I do not know, of course, whether I am absolutely cured or not; it is possible that I may take cold some time and suffer a return of the difficulty. I do not believe it would ever be as bad as before, but if it should come back again I shall take some of Dr. Foo's medicine, which will certainly help me. It has already done me more good than any other treatment that I ever took in my life. It is well for people suffering from chronic difficulties to keep a small supply of the medicine on hand, for sometimes a small dose will prevent a return of the difficulty. For my part I am very glad that I have become acquainted with Dr. Foo's system of medicine.

Yours respectfully, MRS. MALINDA STRONG.
Los Angeles, Cal. August, 10, 1897. 810 West Sixth street, city.

A SEVERE CASE OF ASTHMA RELIEVED.

LOS ANGELES, Cal., October 18, 1897.

I have been troubled with asthma for the past eleven years. During my experience with this disease I have tried every remedy that I have heard of which offered any relief whatever, and have consulted a great many physicians. Nothing did me any permanent good. My trouble was spasmodic in its nature, and all of the doctors whom I consulted informed me that it was incurable. I consulted three physicians in Portland, where I lived for eight years; and five in Los Angeles, all of whom gave the same opinion.

Finally, I went to Dr. Foo, six weeks ago, although I was advised by friends not to do so. At this time I had a most distressing, hacking cough, which shocked all who heard it, and made everyone think I could not live. I was very weak, and the slightest over-exertion brought on a spasm of asthma. I commenced to take Dr. Foo's prescription and my cough disappeared from the first dose. I am now greatly improved in every way. I can take a long walk without fatigue, or without bringing on the asthma. I can also lie down with comfort, as I had not been able to do for years. My appetite, complexion and general health are improved in every particular. I am not yet entirely cured, but the benefit already given me is so very marked that I am entirely satisfied with the treatment, and am confident that I shall be entirely cured within a reasonable time. I knew Dr. Li Po Tai in San Francisco, and I believe that his nephew and son, Drs. Foo and Wing, can accomplish all that the celebrated physiican could accomplish. ANNA ELDER.

617 Montreal street.

Now removed to 623 J street, San Bernardino.

LETTER FROM E. C. WARREN.

REDLANDS, Cal., August 10, 1894.

Dr. T. Foo Yuen, Dear Sir: In answer to your request for a report of my present condition of health; your treatment, my general health, previous and after treatment, it gives me great pleasure to state to you, at present, I am enjoying as good health as ever in my life, or as I could wish to. I am nearly 45 years of age. At an early age I commenced having asthma and inflammatory rheumatism; would have severe attacks of asthma whenever I took cold, which would last me about a week, and rheumatism periodically, about every three or four years, until about two years ago I caught a cold which brought on rheumatism that I could not remove. I was obliged to carry a cane all the time and move around carefully. At about the same time I had an abscess on my lungs and was confined to my bed, and never expected to be better.

Dr. Watrous advised me to go to you for treatment. I at once did so; was examined and commenced to take treatment. This was on the 8th of Nov., 1893. I took about six months' treatment. Those of my friends who knew me before and since treatment say that I am not the same man. I consider you an able physician; your examination by the pulse is simply marvelous. I cannot speak in too high terms of your skill, and shall be pleased to answer any communication you shall see fit to send. Respectfully.

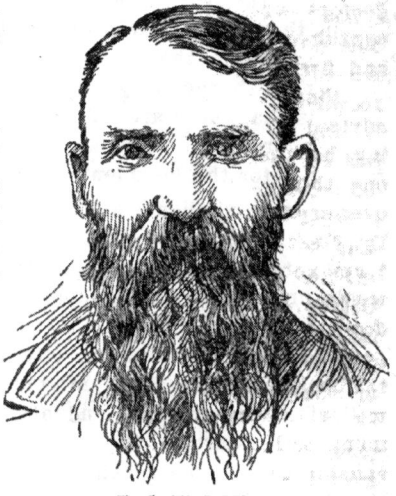

E. C. WARREN.

(Signed)   E. C. WARREN.

Note: Mr. Warren was one of the founders of the city of Redlands; he has been on the Board of City Trustees and is now Justice of the Peace and City Recorder at Redlands. He is a man whose business experience and sagacious nature make it almost impossible for him to be mistaken as to his views, or misled on a subject of such vital importance.

TWELVE CAUSES OF CONSUMPTION AND HEMORRHAGES.

Among the many causes of consumption the following may be noted in this place:

1. Many men and their wives have been poisoned from a resumption of martial relations too soon after the wife has been delivered of a child. At least one hundred days should elapse after child-birth

before the usual relations of man and wife are again taken up. This poison usually settles in the kidneys and weakens them. The system becomes drained of various elements which are essential to the vitality of the person, especially to the health of his nervous system. When these are taken away there is indigestion, which causes inflammation in the stomach. The foods and liquids which should go to nourish the body ferment instead of being digested, and the result is that there are poisonous gases which go through the system and soon reach the lungs. This creates inflammation and affords a good field for the lodgment of the bacillus of consumption.

2. In a similar way venereal poison affects the system, commencing in the kidneys, and afterwards affecting the spinal cord, and passing to the other vital organs. The power of digestion usually yields first and then the lungs become affected, as is shown in the above-mentioned cases.

3. Sexual excesses at any time of life are a fruitful source of consumption. This is one of the most common sources of "quick consumption" and also of "heart failure." The inflammation usually starts in the kidneys and passes from there to the other vital organs, finally reaching the lungs and going through the whole system.

4. Malarial poisoning frequently results in consumption. This may not be the case at the start, because malaria frequently lies in the system for a long time before it breaks out into a severe disease. Then a cold sets the poison in motion, causes fever and often ends in death. It causes consumption by weakening the stomach and and other vital argans. They do not perform their duties properly. Imperfect digestion sets up an inflammation which finally reaches the lungs. A cough is the result and finally a case of incurable consumption.

5. Miners and other persons who are compelled to breathe noxious vapors in underground tunnels or shafts, or in the engine-rooms of steamships or the poisoned air in paint shops, laundries, or dye-houses, or in tenement houses or other closely-confined apartments, frequently become the victims of consumption. In these cases the lungs are poisoned and weakened so that a cold develops into a virulent disorder and kills the patient.

6. Grief, anxiety or intense mental application too long continued will cause consumption. In these cases the circulation of the blood is weakened and the stomach does not receive sufficient blood

to enable it to perform its functions as it should. The nervous system, also, on the health of which the whole body depends, is affected. Imperfect digestion finally affects the lungs and in the same manner as indicated in cause number one.

7. A cold affecting the whole body may settle in the lungs, creating inflammation which will, if not arrested, cause the lungs to fill with phlegm. This hardens and causes severe coughing in the efforts of nature to get rid of it. This coughing wears out the muscles and nerves connecting the lungs and the spinal cord and deprives the lungs of the elements of nutrition which nourish them through the channels of circulation. As a consequence, the lungs waste away and break down and a case of pronounced consumption is the result.

8. A cold which settles in the stomach or the liver.

9. Poisoning through the use of minerals for medication, or for other reasons, such as mercury, morphine, iron, strychine or arsenic.

10. Lack of care during or after child-birth by reason of which there is an incomplete delivery. Portions of the placenta, or congealed blood, are sometimes left in the womb, causing inflammation. A cold which settles in the ovaries, or a cold taken during the period of menstruation may produce the same mischief. The result is inflammation, which finally finds its way to the lungs. The poisoning of the system as a result of miscarriages, whether produced willfully or by accident, is also a similar cause of consumption. Women are sometimes poisoned from intimate relations with men who habitually use liquors, beer, wine or poisonous medicines. Self-abuse, in either sex, is a cause of consumption, producing a weakened state, which affords slight resistance against colds or malaria. The result is a general breaking down, in which the lungs finally participate.

11. Direct injury to the stomach and digestive powers is frequently a cause of consumption. This may be through improper food or insufficient food or over-eating. Taking too much liquid with meals is a cause, or irregularity in eating, or eating nuts, candies, fruit, etc., between meals. Injury to the stomach and digestion soon causes fermentation of the food, as already explained, giving rise to gases in the system which reach the lungs, dry them up, cause them to contract and fail to furnish the necessary vitalization to the blood to keep it in circulation.

12. The habit of chewing tobacco, gum or even toothpicks causes a constant secretion of saliva, which is wasted. The saliva

is secreted by the stomach. There is too great a demand upon that organ, which produces inflammation and an excessive desire for liquids. The stomach is flooded with a supply of cold liquids which it cannot use. Thus the system is weakened, and when the subject takes cold or is exposed to malaria, sickness results which frequently ends in consumption. Smoking also dries out the juices of the system and lays the foundation for diseases of this sort. The difficulty may not be direct in these cases, but they are all bad habits and lay the foundations of many diseases, including consumption. The wearing of corsets is a pernicious habit which often produces consumption in women. This habit will not be discussed at length in this place, but any one who stops to think a little will recognize the fact that an unnatural compression of the body just above its most important organs must sooner or later, give rise to disease and suffering.

Hemorrhages are not always a sign of consumption, although they are often a result of that disease. They may come from the breaking of the small veins in the muscles near the diaphragm, caused by the strain of coughing. Or they may come from the breaking of veins near any one of the vital organs. But they do not always indicate, as many believe, an advanced deterioration of the lungs and they are often much more easily cured than most people think. They yield readily to the herbal treatment when taken at an early stage—before the cough has worn the patient out and perhaps affected the tissues of the lungs themselves.

A CURE THAT IS PERMANENT.

Mrs. M. H. Wilson of Redlands, Cal., was treated by T. Foo Yuen for lung troubles, and cured early in 1894. Her health since that time has been very much improved over her former condition, and she now gives the following statement of her case:

REDLANDS, Cal., September 4, 1897.

The Foo and Wing Herb Co., Los Angeles. Gentlemen: For many years I had suffered from a variety of complications which threatened to end in an incurable case of consumption. I had had la grippe, throat troubles, and my lungs were affected. I took treatment from many physicians in Connecticut, where I was then residing, but all the treatment and all the medicines failed to accomplish a cure, and the doctors finally advised me to come to California. Some time after arriving in Redlands, I heard of Dr. Foo and consulted him. He prescribed for me and placed me upon a diet which, although very plain and simple, accomplished more for me, together with the herb teas, than all the tonics, raw meats, eggs, and other so-called strengthening foods ordered by my former physicians had been able to do.

I was pleased with Dr. Foo's methods from the commencement. His diagnosis was so cerrect that it at once gave me some confidence in him, and the benefit that I received came so soon and continued so steadily that this confidence was confirmed. I was therefore encouraged to continue the treatment for eleven months, at the end of which time I was cured of my lung troubles. This was more than three years ago, and since then, although my physical condition has been delicate and I lack the strength that I had before my first sickness, yet I have been comparatively well and have had no return of the troubles with my lungs. I believe that my cure was as complete as I could possibly have expected, and the long time which has since elapsed shows that it was permonent.   MRS. M. H. WILSON.

A NOTABLE CURE OF HEMORRHAGES.

LOS ANGELES, Cal., October 2, 1897.

The Foo and Wing Herb Co., Los Angeles. Gentlemen: In November last I took a severe cold, which settled on my lungs. My cough became so bad that I was alarmed and consulted a physician, who told me that my lungs were in a very bad condition. I did not feel satisfied with his diagnosis and consulted others until I had consulted six of the best in Los Angeles. They all agreed that I had quick consumption, but none seemed able to help me. I finally went to Dr. Foo and after hearing his diagnosis of my case, I commenced taking his medicine. Within two weeks I was greatly improved and in two months I felt like a new woman. My cough was entirely gone, my complexion had cleared up, and my flesh seemed firm and natural. The poisoned and weakened blood seemed to be removed from my system and to be replaced by new and stronger material. The old blood, from which I received no strength or nourishment, had been made new. I have had no return of the hemorrhages or other symptoms since I ceased taking your medicine, several months ago, and the liver trouble, from which I suffered greatly, has also disappeared. I believe I should have died had I not gone to Dr. Foo just when I did, and I consider my cure the most remarkable, as it has been fully ten years since I have been troubled with this dreadful disease. I have had a great many hemorrhages during that time and have treated with doctors from one end of the continent to the other. Dr. Foo is the first and only physician whoever gave me any permanent relief. I am now entirely free from nervousness and can sleep all night for the first time in ten years, and I feel under the deepest obligation to the doctor for his kind and skillful treatment of me.

MRS. E. ROSS BRITTON,

1025 South Flower street.

RELIEVED OF A COMPLICATION OF DISEASES.

LOS ANGELES, Cal., Sept. 23, 1897.

The Foo and Wing Herb Company, Los Angeles. Gentlemen: In kindly remembrance and acknowledgment of the great skill displayed in curing me of a complication of diseases (among others being kidney, liver and lung troubles,) I now write you to say that I have not felt so well for many years as I have since you cured me of these troubles.

It would be difficult to say in this letter what I have suffered for years from the complaints named above. I assure you for some years I was almost unable to get about, besides I have endured, it seems to me every disagreeable thing that accompanies these complaints, and have scarcely been able to eat anything on account of loss of appetite.

Since the treatment at your hands my appetite has returned and in fact I am a new creature entirely. In acknowledgment of your wondrous skill, and for the benefit of the sick who have no knowledge of the effects of your able treatment, I have written you this letter, hoping it may reach many others, who can be benefited as I have been. Yours truly,

MRS. J. E. BATES,
McKinley avenue, Los Angeles, Cal.

THREATENED WITH CONSUMPTION.

WILDOMAR, Cal., October 10, 1897.

The Foo and Wing Herb Co.:

Gentlemen: This is to certify that I have been treated by the Foo and Wing Herb Company for several months, and I believe it has been the means of saving my life. I had throat and lung trouble and had doctored for years with no apparent improvement. I was told by a Los Angeles physician, just a few days before I went to Dr. Foo that I had only about six months to live and I only went to Dr. Foo because I was urged to by friends; but I certainly have no cause to regret it. Consumption and those diseases of the throat that sooner or later lead to consumption the American doctors do not cure; they only help them for a time. Dr. Foo, I believe, will cure these troubles if the patient will take his medicines long enough and live as he prescribes. IDA RINNE.

APPRECIATIVE LETTER FROM A SAN BERNARDINO LADY.

Mrs. B. Howard of No. 467 C. street, San Bernardino, writes:

"SAN BERNARDINO, Cal., August 6. 1897.

"I feel very grateful for the benefits conferred by Dr. Foo's treatment, not only in my own case, as he cured me of certain persistent catarrhal troubles, but especially in my husband's case. He had been a confirmed invalid for several years, suffering from obscure diseases of the stomach, which had developed a severe cough, from which he was never entirely free. Physicians had cautioned him not to do anything to stop this cough, and one said that nothing on earth could cure it. Two years ago I expected him to die at almost any time. There was, however, a slight improvement, but in January, 1896, he again began to fail.

"About this time I read an article in a daily paper published in San Bernardino in response to an attack which had been made upon Dr. Foo by some of our local physicians. Dr. Foo made a certain proposition, in a very straightforward, conscientious manner, and none of our physicians seemed to dare to accept it. These facts led me to think that Dr. Foo must know whereof he spoke, and, as he was to be in town soon, I was curious enough to go and see him, and induced my husband to go with me, but not expecting to take any treatment.

"While waiting in Dr. Foo's office we met one of his first patients in Southern California, who told us about what had been done for him. This encouraged us. When Dr. Foo made his first pulse diagnosis, it was so correct and satisfactory that we at once decided that my husband should commence to take the treatment which he recommended. In a very short time the change in his appearance was so great that many of our friends observed and spoke of it. He has continued that treatment, at intervals, since that time, with the best of results, so good in fact that he has been able to endure more care and more work in the past year than in the six years preceding, the improvement being a surprise to me, to my husband and to all who have known him."

CURED WITHOUT SEEING THE DOCTORS.

Letters from which the following are extracts have been received from a lady who resides at Bisbee, Ariz., and has been treated by Drs. Foo and Wing by mail, neither of them having seen her. Before she commenced the herbal treatment she was having two hemorrhages from the lungs a week, and has not had one since. Her case had been given up as hopeless by her home physicians. She writes:

BISBEE, Ariz., October 9, 1897.

The Foo and Wing Herb Company, Los Angeles, Cal.; Dear Sirs: I am out of herbs. Would have written sooner, but I was not here in Bisbee. I am improving so fast that I don't like to give the herbs up, for I know that they will cure me. Please send me another month's treatment. I am getting along fast, and a great many people are very much surprised to think that I can be cured.

      Yours truly,   MRS. S. A. KELLEY.

Your letter of inquiry just received. I am mending very fast. My lungs don't bleed any more. My pulse beats 77 per minute as nearly as I can time it. I am still sore and weak in my right side between the top of my hip and the ribs, but not half as sore as I was. I know that your herbs will cure me. My doctors here said the way my lungs bled there was no remedy for me. They may excel the China people in some things, but they cannot excel them in the knowledge of diseases and medicines. I treated so long with our doctors without receiving any benefits that I lost all faith in them, and thanks to the day I saw your advertisement in the Los Angeles paper. May God grant you long life and great success, is the prayer of your faithful friend,   SARAH A. KELLEY.

QUICK CONSUMPTION AVERTED.

SAN BERNARDINO, Cal., April 8, 1897.

It gives me great pleasure to bear testimony to the skill of Dr. T. Foo Yuen, whom I have known for several years, and who has made remarkable cures in the cases of friends of mine, as well as in my own case. I first became acquainted with him on New Year's day, 1894, having gone to see him on behalf of the wife of a friend who was very ill. She commenced treating with Dr. Foo and some time afterwards I learned from her husband that she had entirely recovered, a fact which was a great surprise to me, as I had not supposed that she could get well. This circumstance gave me a very favorable impression of the skill and methods employed by Dr. Foo.

Later I was taken with what appeared to be a very severe cold, resembling an attack of pneumonia, and was for several weeks in a hospital at Riverside, and went to see Dr. Foo. He told me that I was threatened with an attack of quick consumption, but said: "You have come to me in time to save yourself. I will remove the poison from your lungs and in a short time they will grow up and be strong again. My treatment will stop the disease where it is and prevent it from going any farther, and will heal the lungs and cause them to grow again and become as strong as before." I took his treatment for three or four months and the result was as he predicted and promised. I was entirely cured of the difficulty with my lungs, which has never troubled me since. I believe that Dr. Foo's herbal remedies will accomplish all that is promised. Their use involves no nausea or derangement of the digestion or any other disagreeable result, but as far as my experience and observation go they are always beneficial. In many cases they accomplish most wonderful cures. I shall always be grateful to Dr. Foo for what he has been able to do in my own case, and will cheerfully recommend him and the herbal treatment to all suffering people. Respectfully,

J. F. L. M'LAIN.

CHAPTER X.

CURES OF CANCERS, ABSCESSES AND SIMILAR DISEASES.

To tell all about our cures of cancers and similar diseases would require a very long chapter. Even though we gave the full particulars which we have put into our larger book and cannot put into this smaller book, yet we would still not be able to make the subject entirely plain. We shall therefore, reserve this to teach our American students at a later time. Some of the other diseases for which we have remedies are also not explained in this book, and this is for the same reason; because the explanations are too long and difficult for a book of this sort.

We give herewith some account of the famous cure of little Clara Humphrey, which was accomplished by T. Foo Yuen in 1895 and is one of the most remarkable in all the history of medicine. The reader's attention is called to the fact that this case conclusively shows that the herbal treatment is adapted to cases which are supposed to require treatment from a surgeon as well as those cases which would ordinarily, among Americans, be referred to a physician.

We shall give some particulars of this case, in the language of the patient's mother, Mrs. A. Humphrey, who writes as follows:

STATEMENT OF CLARA HUMPHREY'S MOTHER.

LOS ANGELES, Cal., Aug. 19, 1896.
217 East Ann street.

I have a little girl, Clara, now past 11 years of age. About the first of March, 1893, while playing, she fell and bruised her shin bone of the right leg, between the knee and ankle. The injury did not amount to much at first, and for a long time we thought nothing of it. But after some weeks it began to trouble her. I consulted our family physician. He said the injury amounted to nothing and would go away itself. He advised me to rub a little liniment or arnica upon the bruise, which he said would be all that was necessary. Some months later, as the bruise or wound still continued to trouble my little daughter, we consulted another physician about it. As soon as he saw it he declared that the injury was very serious, and asked why we had let it go so long without medical advice, and declared that Clara would be crippled for life, as the limb would have to be amputated. He wanted to perform an operation at once, but we were so much alarmed and frightened that we would not consent to this. We next consulted another doctor, who stated that the injury was more serious than we at first supposed, but that it could easily be cured in a short time. He treated it with liniments and lotions, but these remedies failed to produce the desired effect, and the doctor decided that it would be necessary to open the wound and scrape the bone. An operation of this kind was performed and gave temporary relief, which lasted three months.

At the end of that time the wound again became painful, with a swelling and other indications of a serious difficulty. The doctor now decided that the wound went deeper than he at first supposed, and that a portion of the bone must be removed. So a more radical operation was performed. This operation was performed at the doctor's sanitarium. As I remember there were present eight of the best surgeons in the city. They all agreed in their opinion of the case. They said it was a cancer of the bone, which could not be healed.

They recommended immediate amputation of the leg as the only means of saving my daughter's life.

They thought it would be dangerous to delay this. This opinion was also rendered by other physicians at different times. But the doctor, however, was unwilling to consent to amputation, as he still had hopes of saving the leg. So a section of the bone about two inches in length was cut away nearly to the marrow and removed. After this operation, my daughter was confined to her room for some months, and was not permitted to use her leg at all. But there was no permanent improvement, and the doctor decided that it would be necessary to scrape the bone the third time. This was done about the first day of August last, nearly two and one-half years after the first apparently trifling injury had been received.

Clara grew worse after the third operation and the doctor now declared that, as the wound had not healed, it never would heal; that there were symptoms of blood poisoning and that in his opinion the limb must now be cut off or my daughter would die. He said she could not live forty-eight hours unless this was done. About ten or eleven days after the third operation he came to the house with a carriage, prepared to take Clara to his sanitarium for the purpose of performing the amputation. We objected to this, but he stated that in such cases it was the duty of the physician to overrule the wishes of the parents, who were incapable of forming an unbiased judgment, as he believed, under the circumstances. The doctor had

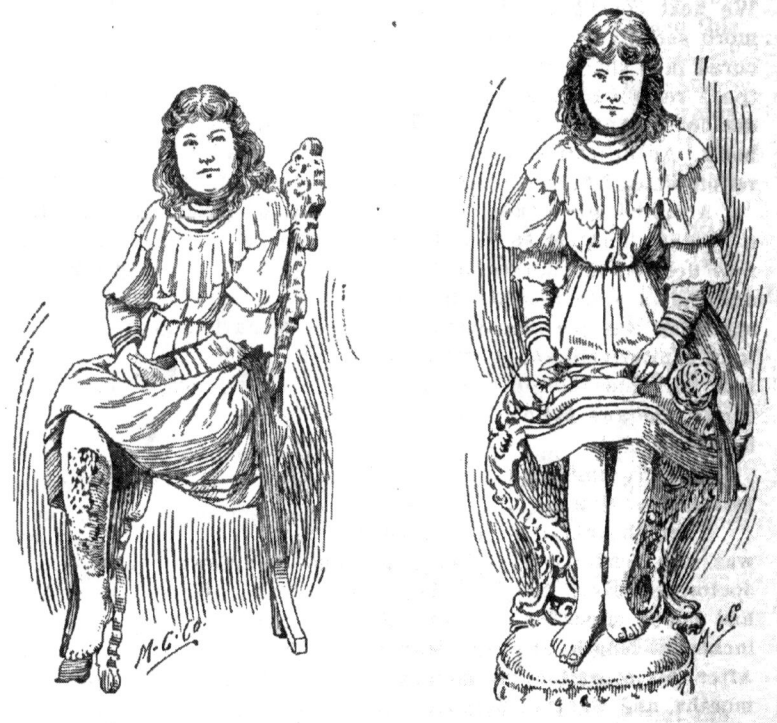

CLARA HUMPHREYS.

been very kind to us and had done everything in his power for our daughter. It was hard under the circumstances to go contrary to his judgment, but I was still unwilling, and so informed the doctor.

Just about this time we began to hear about Dr. T. Foo Yuen through Mrs. Van Luven. Acting on the advice of friends I took Clara to the doctor's office. I was informed by him that the child's system was poisoned as a result of the different operations, and that there was cancer of the bone and no need of an amputation. He said the leg could be saved and my daughter cured, although he predicted that it would take a long time, perhaps a year. I at once commenced preparing and administering the herb teas which I procured from him. I also applied poultices and plasters which he furnished. We continued to use these for about six months. There was a decided improvement in about five weeks, and in about six months we stopped using the remedies, as they were no longer needed.

When we first took Clara to the doctor's office she was so ill and weak that my son had to carry her in his arms. A little later we took her in an ordinary baby carriage. In about six weeks she was able to walk from the street car to the doctor's office, a distance of several hundred feet. In about three months she walked about the house and streets the same as she had done before the injury. She can now walk several miles a day and run and jump the same as other children. There is no limp or other deformity. The injured leg has been completely restored, new bone and marrow having grown and filled up the cavity. She has gained fourteen pounds since using these herbal remedies and is now perfectly well, attends school, and is as active as any child of her age.

I have stated these facts at length because this is the only way to make other people understand the case. Facts speak for themselves and I do not care to add any comment of my own, further than to state that if any people are skeptical as to the truth of these statements they can readily be verified by calling at No. 217 East Ann street. I am, yours very truly.

MRS. A. HUMPHREY.

Mrs. T. Van Luven, a friend and neighbor of the Humphrey family, was the lady who first called this system of treatment to their attention. Mrs. Van Luven was familiar with all the circumstances of this case and gave us a letter confirming the above. It is unnecessary to reprint this letter here, but we desire to give Mrs. Van Luven's name as an additional reference.

CANCER OF THE BOWELS.

The following brief letter from a gentleman in the East who has been cured by the herbal treatment of cancer in the bowels, explains itself. This letter was written after six months' treatment, while Mr. Ingalsbe was in California on a visit.

SIOUX CITY, Iowa, August, 16, 1897.

The Foo and Wing Herb Co., Los Angeles, Cal. Gentlemen: I write you a few lines to let you know how I am getting along. I am a new man from what I was when I first started to doctor with you. The blood and pus have disappeared from the ulcers in the bowels, and my head is clear. My wife says that I would not be alive now were it not for you. I shall certainly remember you to my friends.   Yours truly,

A. INGALSBE.

207 Bluff street, Sioux City, Iowa.
Home address, 366 Bowen avenue, Chicago, Ill.

A CASE SOMEWHAT SIMILAR TO CLARA HUMPHREY'S.

SAN BERNARDINO, Cal., Sept. 27, 1897.

The Foo and Wing Herb Company, Los Angeles:

Gentlemen: About four years ago my son Robert, then 7 years old, received an injury in the hip and knee of the right leg, as the result of a fall. Very soon afterward the bone of the knee commenced growing larger, and continued to increase in size. There seemed to be a great deal of poisoned blood in the knee-pan. It was very hard over the most of the surface, but soft in places. There was trouble with the circulation in the leg below the knee, the foot being, most of the time, as cold as ice. Very soon the boy had to go on crutches, and he continued to use them for years.

I tried various doctors in San Bernardino and Lake counties and they did what they could for the case, but without affording any relief whatever. Some of them wanted to cut the leg off, some called the trouble cancer of the bone, and said it would cause blood poisoning and death after a little unless it was removed. But I was unwill-

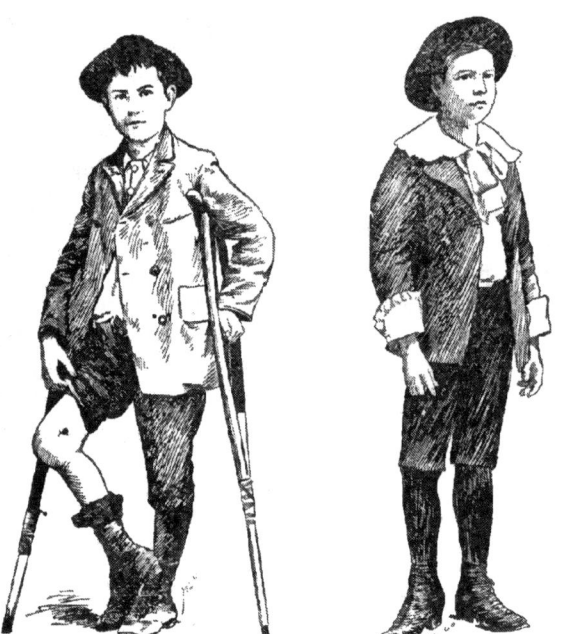

ing to have the foot cut off, and after a while, as the doctors seemed unable to do anything for the case, I stopped consulting them altogether, and tried no more. Time went on, and the knee kept slowly growing worse, and my son had to use his crutches continually.

Finally a friend gave me a copy of Dr. Foo's book, which I was very much pleased to get, as it told about some similar cases which had been cured by Dr. Foo. We went to Dr. Foo, and he commenced to treat my boy. This was in December, 1896. He gave internal remedies and also applied plasters to the knee. After a little there was a great deal of discharge from the knee, brought about by the combined action of the internal remedies and the local applications. Then the knee commenced gradually to grow smaller, swelling reduced 2 1-4 inches in one week, and the medicines also seemed to help the vital organs internally, for the boy's appetite improved, and he grew stronger and had more flesh and a much better color. After one month of the treatment the foot commenced to feel warm and natural, showing that the circulation of the blood had been re-established. Since then he has put away his crutches, except in long walks, after having been unable to go without them for 3 1-2 years. The knee bone is now natural, there is no more discharge and the cure is complete. The boy walks on both feet, the same as anybody, except that there is a little limp, because the right leg is a trifle shorter than the other. This was certainly to be expected after the leg had been out of use for so long, and we are only too glad that the trouble is no worse. We feel that the benefit received has been everything that we could have expected, under the circumstances, and are confident that even this lameness may disappear after a little exercise of the foot. We are certain that no doctor or surgeon could have accomplished more than has been done for this case, and that our boy has been saved from becoming a cripple for life, or, in all probability, from an untimely death.   A. A. DEXTER,

San Bernardino, Cal.

TWO CASES OF CANCER OF THE BREAST CURED WITHOUT KNIFE OR PLASTERS.

The Foo and Wing Herb Company:

Gentlemen: Knowing that there are thousands whose lives could be saved by Dr. Foo, I consider it a duty and a delight to furnish to the world the facts concerning Dr. Foo's marvelous powers in the art of healing.

For a year and a half I suffered terribly, not getting the least relief from the five different highly recommended physicians of Los Angeles, whom I employed. Some treated me for la grippe, others for asthma, one for heart disease. One doctor said my heart was three times its natural size, and out of place; another told me that I could not possible live longer than a year or fourteen months. Surely one could not long endure the ceaseless coughing, the sleepless nights, the unquenchable thirst coupled with the indescribable suffering in the left breast from darting, piercing, cutting pains known only to sufferers with cancer.

When I commenced treatment with Dr. Foo in March, 1894, I had abandoned all hopes of obtaining relief, though I was acquainted with the fact that many wonderful cures had been made by Dr. Foo; still I had my doubts, for I never knew of cancer of the breast being cured; though for over twenty years I was associated with a great many doctors of all schools, while I followed my profession of nurse, traveling with my patients from Canada to the Pacific Ocean. For the treatment of cancer of the breast I have witnessed in hospitals and elsewhere the torturous treatment, and the complete failure of the treatment in numerous cases, and now to be cured by such simple and painless methods by internal treatment alone, places me where I am unable to find language to express my joy and appreciation of Dr. Foo as a physician. I know of another case precisely the same as mine, excepting that the lady had been afflicted longer than I had been. She too has been cured and by the same simple way, and in about the same length of time, eleven months.

Wishing Dr. Foo unfailing strength and a long life, I am an everlasting friend, MRS. JENNIE ROPER.

Station A, Los Angeles, Cal., January 19, 1895.

STRICTURE RELIEVED WITHOUT PAIN.

The following brief letter from a resident of Los Angeles, speaks for itself:

LOS ANGELES. CAL., May 9, 1899.

The Foo and Wing Herb Co., Gentlemen: I am very much pleased with your treatment for stricture, as I am very much benefited without suffering any pain.

Our local doctors could only give me relief by inserting an instrument, which caused a great deal of pain. Yours truly,

C. L. PENSE, 359 S. Olive street.

CASES OF ECZEMA AND THEIR CURES—A DISCUSSION OF THE ORIENTAL SYSTEM OF MEDICINE BY GEO. W. HAZARD—MR. HAZARD'S EXPERIENCE WITH ECZEMA.

LOS ANGELES, Cal., Sept. 3, 1896.

To the Public:

In a former letter, dated August 1, 1894, I said that Dr. Foo had conquered the dreadful troubles I was then afflicted with, and that I had resumed work and was gaining strength every day. After two years I write again to confirm the skill of Dr. Foo and the virtues of the herb medicine. I have not lost a day's work in the past two years, and have not had a return of any of my old symptoms, showing the thoroughness of the cure Dr. Foo made of me. During my sickness my weight went down to 140 pounds, but I soon regained my customary weight of from 175 to 180, and have kept it ever since. At first I followed the diet prescribed very strictly, and I now follow it to a certain extent, although I have found that I can safely allow myself greater freedom in my choice of foods than when I was recovering from my very severe illness. I believe that many things in the plan of dieting are as valuable to the well as to the sick.

I wish to speak of the ecezma from which I suffered in complication with other infirmities. This was so bad that my face and hands were frequently in a perfectly raw condition, like a piece of raw beef, and my eyes were so badly swollen that I was compelled to remain in a dark room and could not use them at all. I was never entirely free from this distressing and painful malady until I commenced treatment with Dr. Foo, but I have had no return or symptom whatever of it since he cured me. This is such a common disease, that I feel sure that many will profit by my experience in reference to it.

My daughter Mabel suffered from malarial poison for a long time. I took her to Dr. Foo in 1894, and after twelve doses of medicine, the poison was completely eradicated from the system, and she gained thirty-five pounds in weight in six weeks, and has continued in excellent health ever since. My other children have also derived great benefit from Dr. Foo's treatment. GEO. W. HAZARD.

AN APPROVED SYSTEM OF MEDICINE KNOWN BY ITS RESULTS. THE ORIENTAL SYSTEM COMPARED WITH OTHERS.

BY GEO. W. HAZARD.

To the Public:

About five years ago the successful medical institution now widely known as the Foo and Wing Herb Company had its origin in an interior city of Southern California. Its beginnings were obscure, but its success was marked from the very first, and its fame soon spread among neighboring communities. Among the warmest friends of Dr. Foo Yuen, who was the founder and is still at the head of this enterprise, are many of his earliest patrons, who received great benefit from his skill in their own cases, and have since watched his career in Southern California with every confidence in his ultimately brilliant success, a confidence which time has fully justified.

The writer was among the earliest of Dr. Foo's friends in Southern California and has watched his career with a great deal of interest. Like scores of others, I consulted Dr. Foo only as a last resort, when nearly dead from a complication of apparently incurable diseases, and after trying everything else in reach. I had the universal prejudice against the Chinese, and the very prevalent notion that their system of medicine is a humbug. I was induced to consult Dr. Foo only by the urgent persuasions of friends who knew something about him, and with very little faith on my own part in his skill, or in the virtues of his remedies. As in hundreds of other cases which I have since observed, I was immeasurably surprised by the termination of my case, for I found myself again a well man, contrary to every expectation on my part, but only after a most heroic struggle on the part of Dr. Foo against the disorders which were threatening my life. Since then I have watched Dr. Foo's progress from an uncertain and comparatively unknown position in a country town to a handsome and well-equipped establishment in the metropolis of Southern California, with a constantly growing influence and a highly satisfactory patronage.

Such an experience naturally sets a man to thinking and the result of the writer's reflections was to change many of his ideas on the subject of medicine. Evidently a cure had been possible in my case, for that was the final result, yet, until I consulted Dr. Foo

I had been going from bad to worse. Nothing had done me any good. Disappointment had followed disappointment, until, weakened in mind and body, I had been almost ready to let go my hold on life. Evidently there must have been some radical and fundamental difference in the methods practiced by my first physiicans and those practiced by Dr. Foo to produce such diametrically opposite differences in results. Under the one regime I sank to the lowest point of my vitality, under the other I gradually rose from that point to a far better state of health than had been mine for years. Now, whence the difference?

In the first place, there was a radical difference in diagnosis. Dr. Foo asked me no questions, except my age. He found out for himself, simply by feeling my pulse, all that he wanted to know, and told me more facts about my physical condition than I had ever known before. Yet every thing that he said was reasonable, and coincided with my experience. A peculiarity of this diagnosis was that it at once gave me confidence in Dr. Foo. I felt instinctively that, if he could learn so much about me in so short a time, by such an examination, he ought to be able to prescribe the proper remedies to cure me. All that was said was stamped with common sense and truth. I did not stop then to wonder where Dr. Foo acquired this extraordinary faculty, but I have since concluded that there is no mystery about it whatever, that it is simply the result of very long and very patient training, based, of course, upon an unusual and inborn aptitude. No one would attempt to make a musician out of a deaf man, and it would be idle to assert that this skill in pulse diagnosis could be acquired by anybody and everybody; yet I am firmly convinced that many could acquire it, perhaps even some of our own white physicians, if they would devote to it as many years of patient practice and as much self-denial in their ways of life, to keep the brain clear and sharpen the perceptions carried from the nerves of the finger-tips to those of the brain, as Dr. Foo has cheerfully devoted. This is too large a subject to discuss in detail in this place. Hundreds have tested pulse diagnosis in their own persons and to their satisfaction, having proved for themselves that it is genuine and philosophical, and the way is open for any other person who desires to make the same test.

The Chinese employ more than 3000 medicinal herbs in their practice. Not one of them is poisonous or injurious under any circumstances. This fact accounts for many of their successes. Their skill in diagnosis accounts for others. Their thorough knowledge of anatomy and of the nature of disease, acquired by vivisection hundreds of years ago, is also a potent factor for success. And their system of diet is the best in the world. They know exactly what foods the invalid should use, and what he should avoid. They have remedies for all diseases, acute or chronic.

There is only one thing for people to do who are in need of help from disease, especially for those who have tried physicians and are still in need, and that is to make a personal test of this matter. This system is now too well founded to be ignored, or to be laughed out of existence, or to be set aside by those who assume it to be wrong, but cannot prove it. It has been shown that its cures are permanent, the one thing that people have been waiting to find out. There can be no doubt that Drs. Foo and Wing have helped a great many people back to a condition of health, out of a most discouraging condition of sickness. Whether they can also help any particular case is a question which can only be determined by a personal interview. The doctors give every facility at their commodious establishment, No. 903 South Olive street, to all inquirers. Everything is perfectly open and free, there is no mystery, no expense. There are plenty of courteous attendants. The best advice that I can offer any invalid is to see Drs. Foo and Wing at once. Delays are usually dangerous. GEO. W. HAZARD.

CURE OF AN OBSTINATE CASE OF ECZEMA.

CEDAR, Ariz., August 31, 1897.

The Foo and Wing Herb Company, Los Angeles, Cal.:

Gentlemen: Although I have never seen Drs. Foo and Wing, yet I have to thank them for curing me of a very obstinate case of eczema. I had been unable to get rid of this difficulty by all the ordinary methods of treatment within my reach, but I had heard a great deal about their cures of other people. I was living in Arizona, and was unable to go to Los Angeles to see them, but wrote to them, and asked them if they could cure me at home. They asked me a great many questions by mail, which I answered as fully as I could. They then informed me that they could cure me at my home. They said "we will change your impure blood and make it new, and you will then be all right." I took a few months' treatment, perhaps three or four, to accomplish this, but at the end of that time I was well. From the results of this method of treatment at a distance, in my own case, I can heartily recommend it to any others who may be similarly situated. I am certainly abundantly satisfied, for it cured me of a very troublesome affliction from which I had suffered for a long time.

WILLIAM P. CARR,
CEDAR, Mohave County, Arizona.

A CURE OF CATARRH AND COMPLICATIONS.

To the Afflicted:

I have been a constant sufferer for over twenty-five years, from the effects of impure water and improper food, carelessness and exposure to the fumes of quicksilver, arsenical and other mineral poisons, while treating rebellious ores. My system had become thoroughly impregnated with them, rendering my liver and spleen inactive, and nearly destroyed my kidneys. Consequently I had dyspepsia, indigestion, catarrh and cramps in the worst form.

For over nine months I could not turn over in bed, without assistance. Two years before that time I could not put on my coat, and four years previously could not ride in the ambulance from Arizona to Los Angeles, on account of the most excruciating sciatic rheumatism, rendering life anything but pleasant.

Though at times in apparent good health, of late years I was threatened with locomotor-ataxia and partial paralysis of my legs, making it difficult and painful to walk, even a short distance, without frequent rests. The cords of my legs and arms had become almost as stiff as steel wire. I had consulted and employed several of the leading and most noted physicians of the day, and had spent hundreds of dollars for patent medicines and other useless,—though much advertised and highly recommended—sure-cure compounds; beside spending over a year at several of the best mineral springs, none of which afforded me more than trifling relief, and I had nearly given up all hope of ever having my health restored.

Fortunately for me, however, I chanced to meet my old-time friend George W. Hazard, who, to my surprise was looking the very picture of health, being the exact opposite of his appearance and condition ten years before.

No doubt, my looks and appearance suggested to his mind his own condition when we parted ten years previously. As soon as I met him he at once began to tell me of his long suffering and almost miraculous cure, which was effected through the skillful treatment of Dr. T. Foo Yuen.

He most earnestly advised, insisted and entreated me to go and call upon the doctor. He said that he used nothing but China herbs to drive out the poison, instead of dosing one with mineral poisons, and apothecary compounds.

But, being exceedingly incredulous, and, in fact prejudiced against Chinese and Chinese doctors in particular, I told him that I would take it under advisement. And, although my prejudice was strong, I could not refuse accepting one of the doctor's pamphlets on his mode of treatment.

The more I investigated "The Oriental System of Medicine," the more I was convinced of its superiority, and of its being in accord with nature.

I at last submitted to being introduced to this most renowned and highly educated Chinese doctor, who carefully diagnosed my case by feeling of the pulse, only. He pronounced my case curable although on account of my age—79 years, and my case being of long-standing and deep-seated, it would take a proportionate length of time to get the poisons under his ontrol, so that they could be driven out of my system, new blood would take the place of old, and nature's recuperating powers would do the rest, and I would be a comparatively well man again, which, I am happy to say after twelve months' treatment, is the case, being free from catarrh, aches and pains. I can now walk miles without resting, and can run up two or three flights of stairs as quick as any young man of my age.

The whole of which I attribute to the skillful treatment of Dr. T. Foo Yuen, corner Ninth and Olive streets, Los Angeles.

I have written this without the knowledge or solicitation of any one. In behalf of those who are afflicted as I have been, I would most confidently advise them to go and see this justly celebrated

Chinese doctor, and be cured. You will not regret the time or expense, or be ashamed to acknowledge that you have done so.

J. C. UDALL,

Los Angeles, Cal., August, 1898. St. Elmo Hotel.

CURED OF CATARRH AND LUNG TROUBLE.

LOS ANGELES, Cal., September 2, 1896.

To the Public:

Dear Reader—I have been troubled with catarrh for several years and for the past two years with lung trouble. I have tried a number of different medicines for my catarrh and lungs, but found no relief until I began taking treatment from Dr. T. Foo Yuen.

I can now say that I feel better than I have for many years. My pains have all left me, and I am not bothered with the catarrh. I feel it my duty to let everyone know what Dr. Foo has done for me. His skill enables him to tell patients, not only their disease, but the causes that lead up to it, and bring on the disease. I advise all sufferers to consult Dr. Foo, and give him a fair trial, and I am satisfied that he will bring them out all right.

This testimonial is sent out willingly and unsolicited in hope that many subjects of suffering humanity may be fortunate to fall into the hands of Dr. T. Foo Yuen, and be so blessed. Yours in sincerity,

C. R. WHEELER.

217 San Pedro street, Los Angeles, Cal.

CATARRHAL DEAFNESS CURED.

LOS ANGELES, Cal., September 4, 1896.

T. Foo Yuen:

Dear Sir: We are very glad to give you a testimonial for our daughter Sarah, who had been troubled with a discharge and deafness of her left ear for the past ten years. Now, after treating with Dr. Foo and taking his herb remedies for seven months, she hears well, has no discharge from the ear, her eyes also have grown strong and her general health is all that we can desire.

MR. AND MRS. W. G. COGSWELL.

FROM A DISTANT PATIENT.

CEDAR, Ariz., August 31, 1897.

To the Public:

Although I have never seen the physicians of the Foo and Wing Herb Company, yet I can cheerfully testify to their success in treating and curing me by means of remedies which they sent by mail and express. I was troubled with impure blood, which brought on inflammation of the bladder, developing into a painful and obstinate case. I knew something about Dr. Foo and his methods of treatment through friends in Los Angeles, who had been among his patrons. One of these is Mrs. Humphrey, the mother of Clara Humphrey, whose remarkable cure is now well-known in Los Angeles. At their suggestion I wrote to the doctors, who sent me the remedies suitable to my condition, as above stated. I am sure, from my experience, that they can make new blood, completely changing and purifying the blood in a person's system, and thus giving health and strength. When I first commenced to take the medicines I felt a trifle bad for a time, but this wore away in two or three weeks, and after that I gained rapidly, in fact at first I gained fifteen pounds in thirty days. All the painful symptoms went away, and I now consider myself as well as I ever was in my life. JAMES WALKER.

CURE OF RUPTURE, CATARRH OF THE BLADDER, SPINE AND KIDNEY TROUBLE, STATEMENT OF C. W. DAVIS.

LOS ANGELES, Cal. September, 1896.

T. Foo Yuen, Los Angeles.

Friend Foo: I never want to lost an opportunity to speak of the good you are doing for the ills of humanity, and of the good you have done me personally, therefore, I make this statement for publication.

I was sick in 1895 for four months, with rupture, catarrh of the bladder, spine and kidney diseases, suffering excruciating pains from failing strength. I had slept but little for three or four months, and was in a wretched condition. I sought the advice of two or three local physicians, who each prescribed for and treated me during the time of my sufferings, but no relief came to me during their treatment. While in this painful and distressed state my friend, Mr. Ditewig, persuaded me to visit Dr. Foo Yuen for a diagnosis of my case, and have him prescribe for me. After taking Dr. Foo's remedies for fourteen days, all my pains had ceased, sweet sleep came to me, my appetite returned, strength and weight increased, while I carefully kept up the treatment for six months, and I became a well man, as I am today attending to my routine business affairs.

I make this statement for publication, with an earnest desire that some fellow-sufferer may be led to see Dr. T. Foo Yuen for similar ailments, or, in fact, any with which humanity is afflicted.

Very respectfully,

CHARLES W. DAVIS.

230½ South Spring street, Los Angeles, Cal.

CURE OF THE MORPHINE HABIT.

SAN BERNARDINO, Cal., October 3, 1896.

To the Public:

Feeling grateful to Dr. T. Foo Yuen for what he has done for me, I wish to say a few words in his behalf.

I have used opium for thirty-two years, having gotten in the habit by sickness, my physician doping me full of it for two years and a half.

When I found out what it was, my system was full of it, and I found it impossible to quit it. I have spent hundreds of dollars to quit the drug, but never could do it. I was failing fast, and if I had not gotten relief I would have been dead long before this. I had often heard of Dr. T. Foo Yuen and his wonderful cures with herb teas. I had doctored so much I had lost all confidence of ever getting relief, only by death.

I thought I would make the last effort. He told me from the first he could cure me, for which I feel grateful, for, of course, I suffered a great deal. I have not used the fatal drug for eight months. Any one reading this, and suffering likewise, may call on me personally, and I can tell them a great deal more than I can write. I live one mile north and three east, on base line, from the city of San Bernardino. Anyone suffering likewise would do well to consult Dr. T. Foo Yuen, as I have the greatest confidence in him and his herb teas.

Yours respectfully,
ABNER McCRARY (aged 66).

FROM A PROMINENT CITIZEN OF LOS ANGELES.

To the Public:

I had been suffering with pains in my kidneys and severe constipation of the bowels for a long time, the result of which was sleepless nights, loss of appetite and rheumatic pains in my feet and legs.

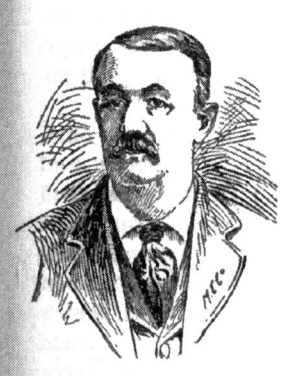

CAPT. C. TAYLOR.

For four months I had rheumatism in my foot, the inflammation was so great I could scarcely put it on the floor, and the swelling extending to my knee joint was so painful I could not sleep. I consulted Dr. T. Foo Yuen and commenced taking his remedies. I felt the effects of the medicine immediately, and I also noticed a marked improvement every day in my condition. I continued the treatment for three months and was entirely cured. My rheumatism was not only cured and the swelling gone, but my blood was purified, brain and nerves vitalized, and the whole system restored and invigorated. I have no pains, my appetite is good, my bowels move regularly and my health is better than it has been for ten years. I am always ready to testify to results and true merit, and I heartily recommend the Foo and Wing Herb Company, No. 903 South Olive street, Los Angeles, to every man who may be afflicted as I have been. T. Foo Yuen has a large practice, and can always be found at his office or a letter addressed to him will have his prompt attention.

I remain your friend,
C. TAYLOR,
520 South Grand avenue.

EXPERIENCE OF A PRACTICING PHYSICIAN.

Dr. B. F. Watrous, of Redlands, Cal., was for many years a practicing physician until compelled by ill health to abandon his profession. In 1893 he became one of Dr. Foo's patients. His difficulties commenced with an attack of la grippe three years before. The final result was chronic indigestion and troubles centering in the liver. He consulted different physicians and spent some time at Bartlett Springs, in Lake county, but got no relief. When he finally returned to Redlands and consulted Dr. Foo, he was suffering intensely from neuralgic pains all through his body and particularly in the chest, back and shoulders. These pains were caused by poisonous gases, which accumulated in the system as a result of its inactive condition. Of his experience with Dr. Foo, Dr. Watrous says:

I met Dr. Foo in July, 1893, and he examined me by the pulse only, saying that I suffered from indigestion, also from liver, spleen and lung trouble. His diagnosis was so perfect that I knew he understood his business, and had confidence in him. I took treatment for about six months, and was surprised to be so much benefited. My wife was taken suddenly ill and died. The shock brought discouragement upon me. I left the doctor's treatment, and took several bad colds, which brought on the trouble anew. At the pressing instance of friends I began the treatment for a second time, and, until this day, have been improving very rapidly.

As far as my observation goes I know that Dr. Foo has perfected many remarkable cures. And I do not know of any case where he has made a mistake in diagnosis or treatment of patients. On the contrary, I have heard his patients say that he always told them how the medicine would act, when they would take effect, and how long the treatment would need to be continued.

I found the doctor a thorough and perfect gentleman, a well educated medical man and a friend to those who suffer. In time his skill will be recognized and sought for even by those who have been opposed both to his methods and to his race. And I believe that his methods and mode of treatment will finally be recognized the world over as the only ones which lead to perfect health.

DR. B. F. WATROUS.

Redlands, Cal., August 8, 1894.

SCROFULA CURED.

LOS ANGELES, Cal., August 12, 1898.

My boy four years old has been ailing for some time, could not eat nor sleep, and suffered from constipation. I was very much alarmed when I noticed a swelling on his neck back of the ear, and decided to take him to a physician. I had read of the cures the Foo and Wing Company had made and I took him there. After feeling his pulse, Dr. Foo told me the trouble was scrofula, and said that he could cure him.

I began giving him the herb teas, and now he seems as well as ever. Has a good appetite and sleeps well. I think the herb teas are good and cannot praise them too much.

MRS. S. A. McINNIS,
1866 East Eighth street, City.

PARALYSIS AND OTHER TROUBLES ALLEVIATED.

LOS ANGELES, Cal., October 22, 1897.

To Whom it May Concern:

For forty years I have suffered from paralysis and diarrhoea. The paralysis was principally in my lower limbs and back. I tried many different remedies, but found no relief, and gradually grew worse until the fall of 1893. During that year at different times I heard of some of the wonderful cures of the celebrated Chinese doctor, Li Po Tai of San Francisco, and thought of going to him for treatment, but concluded that I could not stand the expense of the trip, and—fortunately for me—about that time I learned that Dr. Li Po Tai had a nephew in Redlands who was as skillful and successful in his treatment as the old doctor, and I went from Los Angeles to Redlands to see him.

After taking treatment for some time I was but little better, and had no permanent benefit from paralysis until six months; I then quit the treatment. I did not lose faith in the doctor, as I had much relief from paralysis, and my diarrhea was cured. Something very strange occurred during the next four months after quitting the treatment, at the end of that time I had gained forty pounds in weight, and felt much stronger and better in every way. This reminded me that the doctor had said "That I would gain after I had stopped the treatment."

I get a bad cold occasionally, as most people do, and instead of taking quinine or some other poisonous drug, I go and take the doctor's herbs for a week or two and am cured.

FRANK AMES.

TESTIMONIAL OF A. H. ROSE.

LOS ANGELES, Cal., September, 1896.

Foo and Wing Herb Company:

It is with pleasure I give you this testimonial. I had weakness of the kidneys and bladder and my digestion was very poor. I took your herb remedies for four or five months and my system became cleansed, giving me blood and new life, and I am now a well man.

1032 Blaine street, Los Angeles.   A. H. ROSE.

LETTER FROM A WELL-KNOWN BUSINESS MAN.

Messrs. Wade & Wade are well-known among the business men of Los Angeles, particularly among mining men and all others who require assays of minerals or chemical analyses of any sort. These gentlemen are trained by the requirements of their business to habits of exact observation and close reasoning. It is therefore reasonable to suppose that their opinion is of especial value, even in a matter of professional skill a little outside of their usual line. Mr. E. M. Wade, of this firm, gives the following letter:

LOS ANGELES, Cal., September 5, 1896.

T. Foo Yuen, Los Angeles, Cal.

Dear Sir: I gladly recommend you as a skillful and successful physician, having myself taken your treatment of herb remedies with great benefit. Your herb teas are not only harmless, but beneficial when administered under your skillful direction. Your powers of diagnosis by the pulse, which have been within my own observation and experience, are marvelous. Respectfully,

Chemist and Assayer, 115¼ N. Main. E. M. WADE.

A GAIN OF TWENTY-EIGHT POUNDS.

Mr. W. A. Hallowell, Jr., ex-Deputy Postmaster of Ontario, Cal., and ex-Postmaster of Oberlin, Kansas, says:

I have been in the employ of the Postoffice Department in various States. The steady and confining work brought on my troubles, as I did not take the necessary time to eat my meals—my digestion becoming worse and worse. Indigestion was my main trouble. My kidneys and bladder were affected and everything I tried to do seemed useless. I had been seeking relief and a cure for many years, going to Excelsior Springs, Mo., the Hot Springs, Ark., and Manitou Springs, Colo., also treated with several of the regular physicians.

I came to California in 1886 and to Ontario in 1888. While I was summering in Mill Creek Canyon last year, I heard of Dr. Foo, and, knowing that I had never received any permanent benefits from all the treatment and patent medicines I had taken, I thought that, as he was so famous, he would perhaps help me in regaining my lost health. He examined me, and—impressed with the truth of his assertions as to my derangements—I began his treatment last September. I was down to 95 pounds, and have now gained 28 pounds, and am gaining all the time, even during this warm weather. By following the doctor's diet, I find it to be just suited to my system. I lived up to this treatment and made as good an improvement and showing as anybody he ever treated. I think that Dr. Foo saved my life, for I was extremely low, weak and exhausted. To the sick and afflicted I can cheerfully recommend the Chinese system of medicine as practiced by Dr. T. Foo Yuen. W. A. HALLOWELL, Jr.

Ontario, Cal., August 1, 1894.

CURE OF A FAMOUS ARTIST.

The signer of the following letter, W. G. Cogswell, is one of the best known among American artists, and famous for the many reproductions of his portraits of prominent men, particularly of General Grant. Mr. Cogswell has traveled in many countries, and is a gentleman of wide information and culture. His opinion is of great value. He says:

Having been successfully treated by Dr. T. Foo Yuen for chronic dyspepsia of long standing, and knowing of other remarkable cures effected by him with his herb remedies, I can recommend him to all sufferers as a skillful physician, and a gentleman of rare knowledge and ability. WM. G. COGSWELL,

1138 South Flower street.

Los Angeles, Cal., September 23, 1896.

挨賀惠省蘇華銀行東主前總兵官巴實薦書

BRONCHITIS AND INDIGESTION CURED.

The following letter from a recent patient, speaks for itself:

THE BATTLE CREEK SAVINGS BANK,
ALEX. McHUGH,
　　President;
J. L. RIEDESEL,
　　　Vice-President;
A. BASSETT,
　　　Cashier;
CHAS. WIRTH,
　　　Asst. Cashier.

1723 ROSS STREET,
SIOUX CITY, Iowa, May 10th, 1899.

Dr. T. Foo Yuen, Los Angeles, Cal.—My Dear Sir:

I wish to take this opportunity to thank you most sincerely and heartily for the great benefit which I have received from your treatment. And for the uniform kindness and highly-valued advice, of which I have been the recipient at your hands. I came to Los Angeles with chronic bronchitis of six years standing; extremely sensitive to colds, and every cold taken left me in a worse condition. I had also suffered from indigestion for years, as well as trouble with my kidneys. I was then profoundly ignorant of the existence of reputable Chinese doctors and their remedies. But upon hearing of your great success with hopeless cases, and knowing of no way to procure relief, I concluded to investigate.

Having taken the utmost care that you should have no possible means of knowing anything about my condition, except through your own skill, I found your diagnosis of my case to be so accurate that I concluded to take the herb teas and try the diet. I have never regretted my decision as my bronchitis is, so far as I can judge, entirely gone and I seem to be proof against colds. Neither my digestion nor my kidneys give me any more trouble, and with my weight reduced from 270 to 227 pounds, I feel at least ten years younger and like a new man.

I hope that for the good of afflicted humanity you may continue long in your useful and prosperous career.

Again thanking you for what you have done for me in so many ways, and wishing you long life and happiness, I beg to subscribe myself,

Very truly yours,　　　CAPT. ADAMS BASSETT.

FOO & WING HERB COMPANY

NO RELIEF EXCEPT FROM THIS SYSTEM.

The case of John Scealey, as stated herein by himself, is a splendid illustration of the virtues of our remedies for heart troubles. Mr. Scealey says:

CRAFTONVILLE, Cal., September 2, 1896.

This is to certify that I have recently been a patient of Dr. T. Foo Yuen and have been cured by him of a very long, painful and dangerous illness, called goitre. The circumstances of my case are so remarkable that I feel sure many people will be interested in hearing of them. About two years ago I was taken sick, and was unable to attend to my customary work upon a ranch. I consulted Dr. Foo, who was then living at Redlands, and took two doses of the medicine which he prescribed, paying him for a week's treatment. But so many people called him a fraud, a quack and a humbug, that I was persuaded to let him alone, and stopped taking the medicine after two doses. Then I went to San Francisco and was treated by some of the best physicians there. I remained three months under their care; then, as I was no better, I returned to Los Angeles, and consulted the best physicians I could find there. I was treated for several months by the best physicians in Redlands, and also went to Long Beach, hoping that a change of climate would benefit me, and consulted the best doctors I could find there. All of these changes and experiments did me no good whatever. The doctors all disagreed in their diagnoses. Some called it consumption, but none of

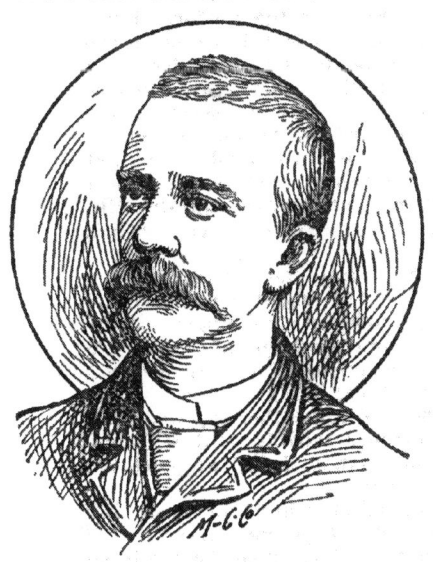

JOHN SCEALEY.

them did me any good. Some of them said that it was enlargement of the heart, and incurable. On the 20th day of February, my physician in Los Angeles advised me to go home, as he said that I could not last twenty-four hours. At that time I had had no rest for a long time, and was burning up with fever which my physicians were unable to control in the slightest degree. My temperature was 106 degrees, and my heart was palpitating at the rate of 140 beats a minute.

In desperation I went to Dr. Foo, whom I had abandoned just two years before for the numerous American physicians under whose direction I had steadily gone from bad to worse. Dr. Foo told me that my trouble was an affection of the kidneys and bladder, which affected the heart, and that the heart case was very much enlarged, causing the goitre. He said that he could cure me, and I commenced treatment. I began at once to get better very slowly, but surely. Within a day or two my fever was less, my pulse was lower and I was able to sleep. In five weeks I went to work for the first time in two years. I continued the treatment for six months, and have just finished it. I am now working every day and feel and look as well as I ever did. It took about three or four weeks to reduce all the swelling of my heart and to take it all away, and to bring my pulse down to its natural beat of 80 to the minute. JOHN SCEALEY.

A WONDERFUL CURE OF HEART AND STOMACH TROUBLE.

BASE LINE, San Bernardino, Cal., September 1, 1896.
To the Public:

I, J. T. Burrows, feel it my duty to say a few words in behalf of Dr. T. Foo Yuen, and for the benefit of any afflicted as I have been. I ailed for many years with pains in the region of my heart and stomach, also with headache in the back of my head and pains in the cords of my neck, so bad at times that I thought I would die. My heart would palpitate until I could hardly stand on my feet. I had doctored a great deal, but had received very little benefit, was very nervous, and I often thought my time had come.

I had often heard of Dr. T. Foo Yuen, and of the wonderful cures he had performed at Redlands, California, so I concluded to investigate his methods. On inquiry I found a number of persons he had cured when they had despaired of ever getting well, having been told by their physicians that there was no hope for them. After taking Dr. Foo's herb teas for three months I gained twelve pounds, and felt well and full of life. Dr. Foo Yuen is a gentlemanly man, in every way kind and courteous, treating all alike.

J. T. BURROWS.

A SERIOUS CASE MADE WELL.

REDLANDS, Cal., July 27, 1894.

T. Foo Yuen:

Dear Sir: If I had any relatives in bad health I should surely recommend them to you. I enjoyed good health until I was wounded in the war of the rebellion. After that I never felt well until I had undergone treatment from you. My digestive organs troubled me always, and, although taking medicines and being treated by several physicians of highly recommended medical institutes, could not get well. A neuralgic pain started in my face, confining itself to my right cheek. The pain grew stronger, and I went to a dentist and had two teeth extracted, but got no relief. I consulted two local doctors, who gave me morphine. I tried another doctor, who during twelve days tried everything which he thought ought to bring relief, but without avail, so I had another tooth pulled. In both instances the teeth were found to be sound.

My mind became seriously affected, and I realized that I was in danger of becoming insane. My friends insisted that I should try Dr. T. Foo Yuen, and I finally consented to do so. As soon as you felt my pulse you said that my case was very serious, adding, "It will be difficult for me to do anything for you; your trouble is caused by the stomach and spleen; I will tell you after ten or fourteen days' treatment whether I can cure you or not." I began treatment. After twelve days you said you could cure me, provided I would follow your directions strictly, adding that the treatment would last about seven months. You examined me day after day, and I improved very much under your treatment. After ninety-four days I became tired of the diet and medicine, and feeling so much better, I thought it was enough, and quit. It did not take me long to see my mistake, and that I had been foolish not to follow on your treatment. You had insisted that I should keep up the treatment three months more, and get entirely well, but I thought it would do, as the treatment had helped me wonderfully; not only did it take that pain away, but did a great deal of good to my general health.

You are a wonderful man and a perfect gentleman and bound to acquire a wide reputation. H. W. TIMMONS,
Notary Public.

MITRAL STENOSIS RELIEVED.

LOS ANGELES, Cal., October 14, 1897.

Some six years ago, while living in Chicago, I began to be ill with what Chicago physicians called mitral stenosis, a disease of the heart. They informed me that the case was incurable, because the mitral valve was closed, preventing the blood from being sent through the arteries, as it is sent in a normal condition, and sometimes, especially under the influence of fatigue or excitement, sending it back into the lungs, causing me great pain and anxiety. I consulted several physicians in Chicago, who prescribed for me. The treatment given was principally digitalis, arsenic, iron, strychnine and similar tonics, intended to stimulate the action of the heart in the hope of strengthening it. I also took a course of baths, devised by a German physician, which were recommended for enlarging the heart, thus giving the mitral valve greater freedom of action. But I received no permanent benefit from any of these remedies and forms of treatment.

Like many others, I came to California two years ago for the benefit of the climate. After residing here for a time I heard of the Foo and Wing Herb Company, and, as a last resort, I commenced to take their treatment. I have continued the treatment ever since, and my general health is improved. I feel encouraged by the results already reached in my case, and shall continue the herbal treatment for another year, the length of time which the doctors say will be required for a complete cure.

MRS. J. PANKEY,
Pico Heights.

A CONCISE DISCUSSION OF ORIENTAL MEDICINE.

SAN BERNARDINO, Cal., October 30, 1896.

To the Public:

My experience with Dr. T. Foo Yuen illustrates some points which I think it is very important that all persons, whether they are sick or well, should understand for their own benefit. I shall therefore make a full statement of the circumstances in my case. In 1892 I commenced feeling somewhat out of sorts, a little different than ever before. At times I was troubled with a feeling of heaviness, which caused me easily to become very tired. Sometimes I had no appetite, and at times I felt slight rheumatic pains coming and going. I was not very sick, but I understood that I was likely to become worse; that there was a root of some disease in my vital organs, which were not performing their proper functions. Therefore I consulted different American physicians for some time, trying to find a medicine that would help me, but I received very little benefit.

This went on until November, 1894, when I became very sick. My feet were swollen very badly. I again took medicine, but became worse instead of better. I had great pain in my swollen feet. I could not sleep and could not walk. At this time I happened to see Mr. James Campbell, who said to me: "Dr. T. Foo Yuen has cured many people whom I know of. Many who have been sick for a long time and have not been able to get help from other doctors have gone to him and been cured. I think he is a man who has had a very good education, and I want you to see him." But I answered him and said: "If the American doctors are so smart and still cannot help me, I don't think the Chinese doctor can do better than they can," and so I did not go to see Dr. Foo.

A GOOD ARGUMENT.

But in March, 1895, Mr. Campbell saw me again and said that if I had taken the white doctor's medicine a long time without benefit and did not try some new way I was very foolish; that this country is still new, and perhaps the doctors have made some mistakes in the methods which they teach; but that China is an old country, and has more people living in it, and that some of those living there must have knowledge, because Dr. Foo had cured lots of patients who had been unable to get any help whatever before they saw him. "It is better," he said, "for you to see him now and not wait too long a time. If you wait too long and become incurable he will not take you." In reply to this argument I said: "I have some well educated friends who tell me that there are some very good doctors in China, but that the Chinese language is harder to learn than that of any other country, and that it is hard to find educated people there. If it is hard to find an educated doctor in China I don't think an educated Chinese doctor would come here; but, as you have talked to me so much about this, the fact does not matter, and I will try to see Dr. Foo," and accordingly I went to see him that same morning. This was early in April, 1895.

TOLD HIM EVERYTHING.

I did not yet believe in the Chinese doctor, but Dr. Foo told me everything about my case without asking a single question except my age. This surprised me very much, and his reasoning about the case convinced me that he understood it. I also saw his certificate from the Chinese Consul at San Francisco and others and from that time had respect for him, and at once commenced to take his medicines. For the first seven or eight days they seemed to make me a little worse, but the doctor told me that they were only stirring up the impurities in my system, and that I should not mind this. In twelve days I began to feel better. I had good sleep and there was less pain. After that I improved all the time until I became entirely well and strong. My skin cleared up and became as white as a newborn babe's in about four and a half months, or one course and a half of the medicines.

HOW TO KEEP WELL.

When I stopped taking the medicine and left Dr. Foo I asked him for directions for following by which I could keep well all the time. I told him I would follow these and take the very best care of myself. He said that in China educated people take care of themselves by stopping a sickness in advance and before it becomes serious. In the summer time they take medicine for five or six weeks and clean out their systems. In the winter time they also take a course of medicine for five or six weeks, and thus they have no sickness, because they keep themselves pure. He said that all persons who have been cured of a long sickness, even though they are entirely cured, nevertheless are not well and strong as young men who have always been well, and that about every six months there is some unavoidable effects upon their systems from different causes. There may be some wear and tear from mental labor, or, as he said, from the seven affections, or the food and drink may not be entirely correct, or there may be some injury from overwork, or some accumulation from the worn-out materials of the body which are not fully eliminated from the system as they should be, or there may be some bad effect from the weather. In these ways sickness comes to all, and one who has been ill is more liable to these attacks than others.

NEGLECT IS DANGEROUS.

If this slight sickness is not stopped then the man becomes worse. The root of the difficulty grows, and by and by perhaps he takes cold or something else is wrong and then there is a bad case of sickness which is very hard to cure and becomes dangerous to life. But if he takes a few weeks' course of medicine summer and winter, twice a year, these troubles are stopped at their commencement, and the man keeps healthy all the time. This, Dr. Foo claimed, was a very good plan indeed.

WORTH REMEMBERING.

I heard what the doctor had to say upon this subject and thought that it was a very good thing for me to remember. After I had gone home the year I was cured I kept improving a long time. I was better all the time until 1896, never being sick at all.

In June and July of this year I intended to take a short course of medicine, but I was very busy, and thought that I could not spare the time. Besides I was feeling so well that I thought it unnecessary to take any more. But between the first of August and the first of October it seemed to me that my system was not in as good trim as it had been, perhaps on account of the long continued hot weather. Then I saw at once what Dr. Foo had taught me was a necessary

thing to know. I made up my mind that it is better to take medicine for health than for sickness. I made a big mistake once when I let my sickness go so long, and do not intend to make another of that kind. I propose to take a short course of medicine for one or two months and to check whatever difficulty there may be right at the start. I can see the consistency and reasonableness of this method and I hope everybody who wishes to take care of his health will give this matter sufficient attention to understand it for himself. I believe that in this way everybody could keep well and healthy, and could stop sickness at the start. As far as I am concerned I will never wait again too long before consulting my doctor, and I believe that Dr. Foo's herbal remedies are the best in the world for this kind of treatment.
E. P. LANE,
With Riverside Water Company.
San Bernardino, Cal., Oct. 30, 1896.
(Witness) JAMES CAMPBELL.

A CURE OF HEMORRHOIDS OF THIRTY-SEVEN YEARS' STANDING—THE CASE COMPLICATED BY INFLAMMATORY RHEUMATISM AND THREATENED PARALYSIS.

Mr. J. W. Symmes is a respected and well-known citizen of Redlands, Cal. He was born in 1830. In early life he was engaged in mining, and contracted the beginnings of his subsequent physical infirmities through exposure in that occupation. His difficulties started with constipation and piles, from which he suffered 37 years with occasional intervals of temporary relief from various physicians. In 1874 a swelling appeared over the short-ribs on the right side, and no treatment could reduce it. In 1889, rheumatism was added to Mr. Symmes' other infirmities, and by Christmas of that year he was absolutely helpless.

Mr. Symmes was then taken to Arrowhead Springs, and took a course of mud baths, with only a slight benefit. He returned to Stockton, and continued treatment with specialists. But he continued to grow worse, and finally went to Redlands for the benefit of the mild southern climate. At this time he was unable to do any work whatever, was constantly in pain, and considered himself likely to die at any time. He heard of Dr. Foo, and consulted him. The results of his treatment by Dr. Foo are best expressed in his own words: "His diagnosis gave me hope, and I was glad to try him. After about five weeks' daily treatment the pain across the back of my head left me suddenly, and I went to look for the swelling which, for twenty years had troubled my side, but it had disappeared; all I could feel was an empty spot and a weakness. While under Dr. Foo's treatment I had to remain on my back for four weeks. I had no more constipation or pain of any kind. Dr. Foo is one of the most conscientious medical men I ever met, and through his skill and the help of God, I have been cured of my ailments of long standing."

The above words were written some three years ago. He has never had a return of his difficulties worth mentioning, and that the cure in his case was permanent as well as satisfactory is abundantly shown by the following letter which we have recently received from him. We offer it as final proof in a case which we consider among the most remarkable of those that Dr. Foo has undertaken. Mr. Symmes says:

REDLANDS, Cal., September 10, 1896.

Dr. T. Foo Yuen, Los Angeles, Cal.

Dear Sir: In response to your inquiry I am pleased to say that my great improvement in health has continued until the present time. As advanced in age as I am, I can now attend to my daily work, and feel well in every respect. In fact, I feel better than I did when I was ten years younger. I am at present engaged in ranching, or some form of out-door work, nearly every day. I consider myself remarkably fortunate in having met you, and become one of your patients at the very critical time in my life when I happened to hear of you. I believe that if I had not obtained relief through your treatment and your herbal remedies, I should not have recovered. I still follow out in great measure the healthy diet which you taught me to observe, and I believe that it is of great assistance to me in keeping my health. I always take pleasure in giving the credit of my cure to those to whom it rightfully belongs, namely, to your skill, efficacious herb teas, and to your system of living.

Very truly yours, J. W SYMMES.

INFLAMMATORY RHEUMATISM RESULTING FROM MALARIA CURED.

I take pleasure in giving my humble opinion of Dr. Foo as a physician. In the first place, his diagnosis of my case, it being by the pulse alone, seemed to me wonderful, he thereby locating my trouble exactly. On my first visit to the doctor I was perfectly helpless, not being able to take a single step without assistance. My legs were swollen to such an extent from the knees to the toes that no joints were visible. This he entirely reduced in five days' treament, and the swelling has not returned in the least. He explained to me the nature of the different poisons in my system and how he would expel them, which he did in fourteen days' treatment. What most surprised me was the simplicity of his treatment and the purity of his medicines, they being entirely vegetable—herbs, roots, berries and barks. This I can verify from personal observation. I am now, after a little over four weeks' treatment, as well as ever, excepting a little weakness in my legs, which are daily improving. My friends who came to see me when I was ill now tell me they never expected to see me out again.

In regard to the success of my treatment, it is more than wonderful in view of the fact that I am advanced in age. I have received treatment from other doctors, but instead of improving I continued to grow worse until I took treatment from Dr. Foo. One who has suffered the excruciating pains from rheumatism alone can imagine the joy of my experience in being cured.

Very respectfully, THOMAS STEWART,
Redlands, Cal., March 1, 1894.

A CURE OF SCIATICA.

LOS ANGELES, Cal., July 22, 1898.

T. Foo Yuen:

I feel so grateful for the relief I have received through your herb treatment that I consider it my duty to let others who are afflicted as I have been know the herb treatment will cure when all others fail.

My complaint was a most severe case of sciatic rheumatism (so called by physicians who treat the effect instead of the cause). I had become distorted and almost helpless before consulting Dr. Foo. In his diagnosis of my case, without asking a question, he pronounced it malaria and mineral poison, which I admitted had been given me as nerve tonics.

Dr. Foo does not treat the effect, but his herb remedies and diet rules have most effectually removed the cause, as well as the mineral poison. Eastern doctors, after months of treatment, sent me here almost helpless. I believe I owe my life to Dr. Foo's herb treatment.

MRS. J. H. SIMPSON,
636 West Jefferson street.

RELIEF OF A VERY DIFFICULT CASE.

LOS ANGELES, Cal., October 20, 1897.

For the past two years my mother, Mrs. L. A. Wright, now 67 years of age, has been confined to her bed or to an invalid's chair with a disease which our family physician called paralysis. It had been coming on by degrees for ten years, and seemed to be complicated by rheumatism, as there was much swelling of the limbs and rheumatic pain. We tried various forms of treatment, medicines, electricity, liniments, etc., without any appreciable benefit. Several physicians declined to treat the case, saying that it was incurable.

Last March we commenced treatment with the Foo and Wing Herb Company. I consider that a complete cure has been made, except that my mother cannot walk yet. The swelling has been reduced, and she has lost some thirty pounds in weight, which was a great improvement in her condition. She can now stand alone, and has the free use of her arms, which she was unable to use for a long time. The trouble now seems to be entirely in the cords and tendons under the knees, which are still stiffened, probably because they have been unused for so long a time; but we are still in hopes that, by further treatment they may become relaxed so as to enable her to walk.

MRS. M. A. WILLIAMS,
1927 Atlantic avenue.

TESTIMONIAL OF MRS. M. D. WERTH.

The following appreciative and kindly letter is from the wife of a well-known clergyman retired from the active duties of his calling and residing in Los Angeles. Mrs. Werth says:

I feel it my duty, for the encouragement of the sick and suffering, to give my testimony for what the Foo and Wing Herb Company have done for me.

When I moved with my family from San Francisco to San Diego, I began to feel sick. I was unable for some time to superintend my household, until I was stricken down with la grippe of the worst kind. For a while my friends feared for my life; I became so weak that I was unable to move or rise from my bed without assistance. It seemed that I had only a few more days to live, and even my physicians despaired of my recovery. After a long spell of sickness I recovered slowly, but found that, while la grippe itself had left me, there remained a continual pain in my back, which almost disabled me to do any work. I tried several remedies, but in vain. I consulted different physicians, but they gave me no permanent relief. I feared that other complications might set in, and soon experienced kidney trouble, feeling weaker every day, and had a continued feeling of tiredness.

When Doctor T. Foo Yuen and his associates moved in our neighborhood, I noticed that very many sick people came to the doctors for treatment. When I inquired of some of them as to the efficiency of their remedies, I heard nothing but praises, and some of them testified as being cured entirely and permanently from diseases that seemed to be incurable. This caused me to visit the doctors.

To my great astonishment, the doctor asked me no questions, but after he had felt the pulse of my right and left hands, told me all about my maladies, even locating the pains in my back so plainly that I could not have described them any plainer. It was perfectly natural for me to think that a doctor who knew my sickness so well would certainly know the remedies for the same as well.

After taking a few doses of his medicine, I felt a change for the better, the pain became less severe, the tired feeling left me, I became more cheerful, and now I am entirely well, joyful and happy.

I have written these lines to express my gratitude to the physicians of the Foo and Wing Herb Company, and to recommend them to the sick and the afflicted as most skillful physicians.

MRS. MARY D. WERTH,
916 South Broadway, Los Angeles, Cal.

NEURALGIA CURED.

406 Mason street,

SAN FRANCISCO. Cal., March 24, 1894.

To Whom It May Benefit:

I do willingly add my endorsement to the superior skill and excellent faculties of Dr. Foo in handling diseases of all natures and stages. I would certify that, during the summer of 1893, while at Redlands, I was taken with a severe attack of neuralgia, which I supposed originated from a decayed tooth, but which idea I abandoned, after having the tooth extracted. I would writhe in misery from midnight to sunrise. I consulted Dr. Foo, who diagnosed my case as arising from malarious gases in my system. I began treatment, and in two weeks' time was so benefited that the attacks were less severe and changed to the forenoon. At the end of the eighth week I was entirely cured. The effect of his medicine was such that it not only affected the local symptoms and seat of disease but acted on the whole system, thereby causing me to feel healtheir than ever before.

I would also add that during my acquaintance with Dr. T. Foo Yuen I have always found him a most estimable man and a perfect gentleman, who never offended anyone, being always of a genial disposition and thoroughly intellectual. This testimonial is sent willingly and unsolicited, in hopes that many subjects of suffering humanity, who may be so fortunate as to fall into his healing hands, may be so blessed.   Yours in sincerity,

(Signed)   EDWIN CAMPBELL.

CURE OF BRAIN FEVER AND OTHER DIFFICULTIES.

R. D. Brumagim of Redlands was treated by Dr. Foo for brain fever, and afterwards for other difficulties less severe. Of the results of the treatment in his case he speaks in the following appreciative language:

REDLANDS, Cal., January 18, 1895.

To the Public:

I can speak in very high praise of the skill and knowledge of Dr. T. Foo Yuen. The remarkably short time required to give me complete relief in three different attacks of intense suffering—one of brain fever, from which I recovered to resume my business duties in ten days—and the other troubles being completely removed with only three and five doses of medicine, is convincing evidence that Dr. Foo's medicines are in perfect harmony with the laws of the human system. Such immediate relief could be afforded only by a selection of the proper agents, and as a result of a positively correct diagnosis.

When I review in my mind the many complete cures that Dr. Foo has effected, in cases which were considered incurable, and doubtless were incurable by other methods, I am led to hope that the day is not far distant when his system of medicine will be adopted generally. R. D. BRUMAGIM.

CHAPTER XI.

THE CAUSES AND CURE OF PILES.

Piles, or hemorrhoids, are called by many different names. The term hemorrhoids is properly applied to all of the different forms of this disease. In extreme cases the trouble takes the painful form of a fistula. There are blind, bleeding and itching piles, inward piles and outward piles, but all of the different kinds arise from similar causes.

If the piles are external they are easily cured by the use of our powders and ointment. But those that are internal and cannot be seen are more difficult to cure because they are harder to reach. Still, if one has the proper remedies there is no difference in the end between the hard and easy cases. They can all be cured, provided that the remedies can be made to reach them, and we have remedies which can do this. The causes are the same and the remedies are equally good. The only difference is in the method of application.

Some cases of piles arise from the use of improper foods and liquids. This gives rise to poisons resulting from indigestion and fermentation of the food in the stomach. The poisons settle in the intestines, and, every day, when the bowels move, the poisons are forced down into the rectum, and, little by little, in the course of time, the piles take form. Piles cannot arise at once, but come by degrees in the way just stated. Some piles are caused by malarial fever, which is improperly treated by poisonous mineral remedies. These accumulate in the bowels and cause piles, after a time. Some cases arise from syphilitic poison, which is thrown off from the kidneys. When mercury is taken for the cure of syphilis piles are often caused.

Some physicians cut the piles away and cause them to discharge from the inside. Sometimes inflammation from the lungs passes down through the intestines and causes piles. The lungs and the large intestines are connected, and what affects the one will affect the other. Some cases of piles arise from dysentery, or bloody flux, which is improperly treated. The mucus arising from it is not taken away, because condensed medicines are used which stop the movements too quickly. The impurities thus left in the system settle deep in the rectum and a case of hemorrhoids is the result. Measles and some skin diseases produce piles when the poison resulting from them is not fully removed. Sometimes, in cases of childbirth, all of the congealed blood resulting is not removed and causes piles by finally settling in the rectum. Sometimes blood poisoning acts in a similar way. It sometimes attacks the muscles of the lower bowel and causes a running of blood after the movement of the bowels. Sometimes poisoned blood arising from the stomach or kidneys, when diseased, settles in the rectum and causes itching piles. The liquor habit causes piles. So do certain other diseases of long standing. In like manner sometimes the pile poison causes other diseases, if it is not removed from the system for a long time.

In this way many different things cause piles and the root of the poison is very deep-seated. It goes along the kidneys, intestines and stomach. Sometimes it arises in the womb and goes through the womb, the kidneys, the ovaries and the bowels. This congealed blood remains in the body so long that its being there is a sort of second nature and it goes all through the vital organs. It is necessary to use internal remedies in order to remove the root of the poison. Also to use external remedies, such as our powder and ointment, in order to draw away the poison from its deepest location and to get rid of it through the outside of the piles. This process causes the piles to swell for a few days, while the poison is gathering in them. Then they begin to discharge and the swelling goes down. The piles grow smaller and soon disappear entirely. This is certainly the very best way to treat this disease in any of its forms, because there can be no permanent cure unless the poison is entirely removed from the body.

The most difficult form to treat is that known as inward piles. In these cases there is much suffering after every movement of the bowels. Internal remedies are required to cure this form of disease and also our steam treatment and some of our injections, which carry the remedies directly to the seat of the trouble. These remedies are invaluable in these forms of disease. Every time they are employed the fragrant smell from them fills the room, and from this you will know that they are very good as well as strong. But both forms of remedies, the internal and the external, must be employed in order to get the full benefit. Sometimes persons afflicted with this disease employ physicians to cut the piles away. But if they do cut them away they still do not cut away the root of the disease. After a few months the trouble comes on again as bad as ever, or worse. Cutting affords no permanent cure and the patient finally has to come to us. It is much better to come to us in the first place and save the pain and suffering and delay of these unprofitable operations. To remove the root of the trouble is the only possible way of effecting a cure.

The Foo and Wing Herb Company has always followed the above methods and has accomplished many cures. We have even cured cases where there have been abscesses in the bowels or liver or even cancers. The treatment for inward piles will cure all these troubles. We have had so many testimonials of these diseases which have been cured that we cannot print them all. We give you the testimonial of Mr. Symmes, for instance. He suffered first from piles, which were not cured. Afterwards this became rheumatism. G. W. Hazard was ill first from eczema and paralysis and these afterwards developed into piles. The case of Sadie McPherson of Santa Ana was similar. So was that of Mrs. Hendrickson of Redlands. She had difficulties of this sort which we cured at Redlands, but her testimonial does not mention the piles because her principal difficulty was from another disease. Our book contains many testimonials of this sort, where this disease was complicated by others.

But all of these used the same treatment to draw the poison from the system. The testimonial of Mrs. Shevan, in this book, is another example. She called her malady an abscess of the liver and bowels, but we employed the same treatment to draw away the poisons and impurities which were causing the abscesses. A similar case was that of Mr. Ingoldsby of Chicago, who was treated for cancer of the bowels. We employed the same treatment. By these illustrations you will understand how diseases that are called by different names and, in some respects, have different symptoms and afflict the patients in different ways, are really from the same or very similar causes and may be cured by the same treatment. The blood must be purified by internal treatment and external remedies must also be used, these being varied to suit the needs of different individuals. But we have been uniformly successful in all of these very painful, and, if neglected, dangerous diseases.

SHORT AND TO THE POINT.

SPOKANE, Wash., Oct. 15, 1898.

The Foo and Wing Herb Company, Los Angeles, Cal.:

Gentlemen: I take pleasure in testifying to the remarkable curative virtues contained in the remedies used by you in your practice. And also to the successful treatment and skillful diagnosis of the most stubborn and difficult diseases. My wife had been a sufferer for many years from bronchial catarrh and piles. Had been treated by the best specialists in various cities without any benefit. But under your treatment was entirely cured of piles in a few weeks, and has been greatly helped in her bronchial trouble. I would cheerfully recommend all sufferers to consult these educated gentlemanly Chinese physicians, knowing that they will do all that human skill can accomplish.

Gratefully and truly yours, V. C. MILLER.

I fully concur in all the above.

MRS. V. C. MILLER.

PILES, CATARRH AND GRANULATED SORE EYES COMPLETELY CURED.

State of California,
County of San Bernardino.

Newport Lumber Co.,
REDLANDS, Cal., Feb. 25, 1894.

T. Foo Yuen:

Dear Sir: In regard to your inquiry concerning what benefits I have received under your treatment, I would say first, by way of explanation of my troubles, that I had what is commonly called blind bleeding piles, also catarrh and granulated eyelids, all of which have bothered me for years, and for which I had, at different times, doctored with five leading physicians of Southern California. The first trouble mentioned had become of such a painful nature that I was told that nothing but an operation would ever relieve me, and the chances of it not being successful were not pleasant to contemplate. As to my catarrh and eyes, I was under the direction of a physician, treating them daily. Through friends, I had heard of your wonderful power in diagnosing, and some cures you had performed, although you had but recently come to our city.

I tried to smother what prejudice I had for the "heathen," and was driven up to your office for treatment, after which I was thoroughly satisfied, for without a word from me—through the pulse alone—you told me exactly my trouble and its cause. While the cause was to me entirely new, the reasons given were so practical that no one could help but believe them. I commenced a course of treatment, going to your office nearly every day, and am now—at the end of five months—entirely well of my ailments.

Yours very respectfully, G. E. FOSTER,

Subscribed and sworn to before me, this 12th day of April, 1894.

(Signed) FRANK C. PRESCOTT,
Notary Public.

CURED OF A COMPLICATION OF DISORDERS.

SAN BERNARDINO, Cal., May 29, 1897.

As the proprietor of the Occidental Hotel in San Bernardino, where Dr. Foo had an office at intervals for two years and a half, I had a chance to see very many of his patients and to watch the effect of his treatment. At first I had no faith whatever in Chinese medicine, and, although I had been suffering for a long time with bowel trouble, I would not consult Dr. Foo.

I noticed that nearly all the people who did consult the doctor were afflicted with old, chronic diseases, which were very difficult to cure, and I supposed that most of them had been given up by other physicians. Very much to my surprise I found that they all got along nicely, and I began to hear them tell about their cures and to praise Dr. Foo and his remedies.

All of the cases got along so well that I became satisfied to take the treatment. I had already tried several different physicians and had received no benefit. My general health was very poor then, as a result of my bowel trouble. I had no strength and wanted to lie down all the time. I also had fever much of the time, and stomach and bowel trouble all of the time. I commenced the treatment, and, after one month, began to see a benefit from it, and after that I improved all the time, and after two months I looked very different than I had before. I grew stronger, had more energy, and wanted to do something. In three or four months I was completely cured, and have had no return of my difficulty since then. My health is now so good that I realize the great benefit which I have received, and wish to say something for Dr. Foo, so that other people who are afflicted as I have been may also have an opportunity to be cured.

MRS. E. R. VAN DEURSEN.

TESTIMONIAL OF MRS. HENDREN.

LOS ANGELES, Cal., November 25, 1898.

The Foo and Wing Herb Company:

Gentlemen: My recent experience with your remedies in a case of diphtheria is well worthy of remembrance.

I took a severe cold, with light fever and great pain in my throat. I was confined to my bed at once. After a few days the throat difficulty grew much worse. My friends thought that I had diphtheria.

I had heard of the wonderful cures effected by your Company, and I was acquainted with Mrs. Werth, one of your patients.

My daughter called on doctor Foo who gave her one of his question-blanks. I answered the questions and he sent me remedies. He said that I was surely threatened with diphtheria, and had got the remedies just in time to arrest the attack. I took the remedies and was able, in a few days to leave my bed. I am sure that these remedies saved my life.

I continued the treatment for one month, and have since felt better that at any time for the past ten years.

Very truly yours, MRS. BELLE HENDREN,

S. Hill street, cor. Sixth, "Norwood."

AN ATTACK OF DIPHTHERIA AVOIDED.

LOS ANGELES, Cal., April 18, 1897.

Last February my daughter Lulu went through a severe attack of la grippe, which was followed by complications that threatened diphtheria. Her throat was very badly swollen; she had a high fever and was unable to leave her bed for a few days. The physicians of the Foo and Wing Herb Company commenced treating her at once. The treatment consisted of the herb teas and of powders which were blown into the throat to prevent the formation of the ulcers which usually appear in cases of this kind. My daughter was out of bed in two or three days and able to go out of doors as usual in a couple of weeks, although she was a long time in recovering from the weakness brought on by the sickness. She has had no sore throat or any trouble of the sort since.

Dr. Yoth, who happened to be at the house during this illness, and saw my daughter several times, said that all of her symptoms were those of threatened diphtheria, and that if it had not been for the prompt and effective treatment given her it would undoubtedly have gone forward into a severe illness, which might have endangered my daughter's life. We considered ourselves very fortunate in the termination of the case, especially as there were no after effects, which so often follow cases of this sort and are often of great injury to the health for many years or for life. The herb teas prevented anything of this sort. MRS. M. A. HAZARD.

THROAT TROUBLES AND COMPLICATIONS—A VARIED EXPERIENCE.

REDLANDS, Cal., April 30, 1897.

To Whom It May Concern:

My acquaintance with Dr. T. Foo Yuen now dates back about four years. It commenced when I consulted him for different difficulties which had troubled me for a long time, finally taking the form of so-called bronchitis, with ulcers in my throat, pains in my chest and a general debilitated condition. I had also been greatly afflicted with hemorrhoids.

Dr. Foo informed me that all of these difficulties had their origin in a poisoned condition of the system, dating from the birth of my son, thirteen years before, and that if they were neglected, as time went on, they would grow worse and might result in rheumatism or consumption. His pulse diagnosis was so complete that I was both surprised and pleased. I commenced treatment, and in about four months was completely cured. I became in every way better and much stronger than I had been for many years.

As I lived next door to Dr. Foo for two years in Redlands I had opportunities to know many of his patients, and I also afterwards tested his methods of treatment when my children were ill, once with a case of scarlet fever and once with la grippe. I learned to respect Dr. Foo thoroughly as a physician and to honor him as a man, for his uniform courtesy and kindness of heart, as well as for his great skill and his many successes in very difficult cases.

As time passes, although the doctor has removed to Los Angeles, I have still known of him, and have heard with pleasure that his practice has steadily increased and that his reputation has grown greater year by year. I believe that the more widely this system of medicine is known the better it will be for American people. During the four years which have now elapsed since I was cured, my own health has been so good, as compared with what it was before that, to my mind, the value and permanency of the cure possible through this system of medicine are established beyond a doubt. I shall always consider it the very best way known to man of treating all disorders of the human body.

One other thing I wish particularly to mention, as it may save some one else from a great deal of suffering. Last September I was bitten on the arm by a black spider. I called one of the best physicians in Redlands, who did everything in his power for me, and probably saved my life, but he told me frankly that he could not remove all of the poison from my system and that I must outgrow it. The veins turned black all over my body, and I had, day and night, indescribable pains resembling those from acute rheumatism. I had no relief from these for ten days, and looked at the end of that time like a person who was just recovering from typhoid fever. Dr. Foo then came to Redlands, and I consulted him. In a very few days after taking the herbs that he gave me the pains all left me and I gradually recovered, although it was several weeks before I had my health back again. The bites of these spiders are sometimes fatal, and I consider myself very fortunate in knowing of Dr. Foo's skill and in being able to avail myself of it at this time.   MRS. A. J. HENDRICKSON.

MEDICINE VERSUS SURGERY.

Growth of a Popular Fad for the Use of the Knife—Thousands of Unnecessary Surgical Operations—Nothing Impossible With the Proper Remedies—A Case that Completely Proves the Value of the Herbal Medicines.

The human mind is the most perverse thing in the universe. Everything else is governed by invariable laws, but the freedom of action permitted thought also permits mankind to deviate, to a certain extent, from the natural laws provided for its benefit. Man may do as he chooses in many things, and he often abuses this liberty by choosing to act against his own best interests.

This is emphatically true of everything relating to the laws of health. We do what seems agreeable, regardless of the consequences. When baleful results of our course of action compel us to reform and to seek relief in medical treatment, we still get as far away as we can from the simple processes of nature. Our methods of medical practice are artificial. They do not conform to the processes of nature as seen in the growth of all forms of life, vegetable and animal.

These are replaced by the devices of human ingenuity, which appear to be reasonable, but are unsuccessful because they are not in harmony with nature. Modern surgery is an especially conspicuous example of great skill and the highest technical knowledge misdirected and misused. It is a glittering fraud because its methods, which compel admiration by their brilliancy, are nevertheless destructive of health and do not accomplish cures.

ONLY ONE METHOD OF CURE.

In a broad and general sense there is only one method of curing disease and that is nature's method of growth and change from within the body. The method of growth is also the method of cure. A diseased portion can be replaced by a portion that is sound by the same process of growth which originally created it—provided that it can be fed. This is just as true of the tissues of the brain or of the bone as it is of the skin or the flesh. The whole secret of success in the treatment of any disease is in furnishing the body with the proper food through the stomach and the blood. This may be assisted in many cases by outward applications to heal those tissues that have become inflamed and to remove those that have been destroyed by the progress of the disease. In these cases success comes from a skillful use of both internal remedies and external applications.

NO BRICKS WITHOUT STRAW.

The skill of the best workman is unavailing if he has no tools and no material to work with. Yet the modern physician, who is supposed to be a workman of the highest skill, selects the poorest tools and the worst materials within his reach and attempts to bring about the most important results, depending upon the most intricate processes. This is a most curious and astounding exhibition of illogical reasoning, yet it is seen every day in every civilized community. Apart from accident and external causes disease usually results from the presence of some poisonous substance in the blood, creating inflammation, from pressure upon or other derangement of the nerve centers, from failure of a vital function, or from lack of nutrition. To remove or remedy these conditions the average physician goes directly away from nature's methods and selects poisons which he administers in the place of foods. When he desires immediate results he injects these directly into the blood, employing a degree of haste and force which is in itself contrary to nature and productive of great injury. When he attempts to feed a patient, who is starving in the midst of plenty, because he cannot properly assimilate his food, the modern doctor overdoes the business by administering the richest and most concentrated foods within his reach, forgetting that all processes of growth and healing are necessarily slow and cannot be hurried.

THE FOUNDERS OF A BETTER SYSTEM.

The one nation that has consistently followed a better system than this for hundreds of years is one that is little known and often misunderstood. Yet it has given to the world many inventions of incalculable value. It originated the art of printing, which is the foundation of all modern civilization. It invented gunpowder, upon the use of which are based all the gigantic and complex results of modern warfare. In the fine arts it has produced the finest papers, the most delicate tapestries, the most cunning products of metallurgy, the most beautiful results of the potter's skill. In all these lines it preserves secrets that are centuries old, yet they accomplish results that cannot be improved upon. They embody the whole sum and substance of human knowledge upon these subjects. The same fact is true of their medical system. It is not to be despised because of its antiquity. On the contrary, its consistent use by a great and constantly-growing nation, for hundreds of years, proves its superiority over our own, which is constantly changing but never improving.

THE CHINESE HERBAL SYSTEM A SUCCESS.

The Chinese herbal system of medical treatment is a success. Facts speak louder than words; results are better proof than theories. Experience must and will finally overcome prejudice. Every patron of this system is a living advocate of its merits. The number of these is constantly growing. They quietly recommend this system to their friends, and every day some timid and unbelieving invalid gathers courage to test the system in his own case. The results in scores of cases surpass the highest expectations of those who enter upon the treatment. Every now and then some cure is accomplished that is especially brilliant and astonishes even those who are familiar with what this system of medicine can do. It cures because its methods are based upon the methods of nature—the real healer in every case—and have been perfected by centuries of experience.

BETTER CURE THAN CUT.

By a modest estimate, the herbal treatment would cure 50 per cent. of the cases that find their way to the surgeon's operating table. And it is to this phase of the subject that we desire to call attention in this article. It is certainly one of the most important open to public discussion, for no one can tell when accident or disease may render it of special importance to himself or to some member of his family. To be forewarned is to be forearmed, and some of the people who glance at this article today may be glad to remember it a year from now. This has been our experience in the past, for facts and illustrations of cases that were put before the public long ago are still bearing fruit and doing good by informing the afflicted where relief may be obtained. Most people are careless of their health, but some have the good sense, after they have lost it, to seek for the best means of regaining it. We have had the pleasure of assisting many of these and hope to assist many more.

THE ORDINARY ROUTINE.

The average practitioner of the day dislikes cases that may call for surgical interference. He knows that he cannot cure these with the remedies and the skill at his command. So he refers them to the specialist, a physician who is supposed to have made a special study of a number of diseases and to have unusual resources at his command for curing these, because he limits his practice to a few. But the specialist, although he may know more in his line than the general practitioner who distributes his energies over a wider field, has only the same remedies at his command. He may use these more intelligently in certain cases, but his resources are nevertheless limited. We will admit that he sometimes cures, but when he fails, as he often does, there is then only one other thing to be done. That portion of the body which is diseased and cannot be healed must be cut away. This is the surgeon's opportunity. An operation is performed and the patient is maimed, to a greater or less extent. He is not cured, but he is usually thankful for escaping with his life. Often his health is wrecked and he becomes a confirmed invalid as a remote consequence of the operation, but he usually believes this to have been unavoidable and so drifts along thinking that he has fared as well as he could have expected.

THIS IS A MISTAKE.

There are hundreds of cases where all this misery and suffering and resulting sickness is unnecessary. In these cases the operations could have been avoided and the patients could have been restored to health without suffering or danger of any kind. There are scores of men and women in Southern California today who are congratulating themselves that they escaped the direful results of surgical operations through the Oriental System of Herbal Medication. This is especially true of many women, for in the field of the diseases of women the specialist and the surgeon find their golden opportunities. Many of the cures that we have made are unknown to the general public, although we know that those who have been cured are very grateful to us. A few have been so remarkable, so absolutely unprecedented, that we have felt justified in placing the details before the public. These have aroused a great deal of attention and have excited much discussion, which has done good because others who needed the benefits of our skill have heard of it. One of the most remarkable of these cases was that of little Clara Humphrey, who was cured by us in 1895. After two years of incessant suffering and three unsuccessful surgical operations, we took her, at the last moment when eight leading surgeons of Los Angeles declared that amputation of her leg was necessary in order to save her life, cured her and restored her to as perfect a condition of health as she had ever known, without lameness or any deformity. Another remarkable case was that of Robert Dexter of San Bernardino, who suffered for three years with lameness resulting from a trifling injury to his knee, which was not properly treated and went from bad to worse, until it became a deformity that was chronic and even threatened his life from blood poisoning. We restored him to health and the activity of youth after every other means had failed. We mention these cases especially because they were chronic diseases of the bone and the popular, though utterly false, idea is that these cannot be successfully treated by internal medication.

ONE OF OUR REMARKABLE CURES.

SAN BERNARDINO, Cal., August 5, 1898.

T. Foo Yuen:

I feel so truly grateful to you for the wonderful cure you made in my dear child's case, that I cannot refuse you a testimonial. Six years ago my son, Roy E., then three years and a half old, was thrown from

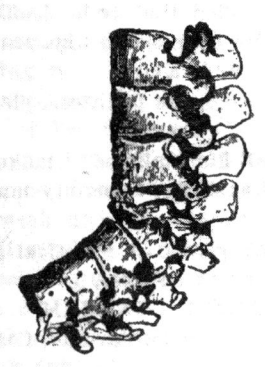
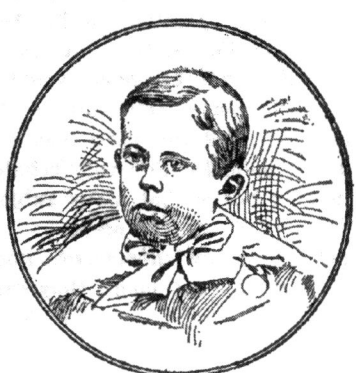

ROY E. BURCHAM.

a hammock and injured his spine. Soon after an enlargement was formed. The first doctor that I consulted informed me that the vertebra did project in that way sometimes, and that was nothing to worry about.

As he grew worse, I consulted another doctor, and he immediately put on a plaster-paris jacket. In about two weeks an abscess broke under the jacket at the point of injury. As he was such a healthy child, that soon healed.

Six weeks from the time the first jacket was applied, a second one was put on, and in another six weeks he underwent the torture for the third time. He suffered so much that the doctor soon removed that and found that another abscess had formed lower down, and at the side of the spine. That was called a "cold abscess," and was allowed to get "ripe" and when it was opened a pint of pus was taken out, and in three weeks' time half that quantity. Then a drainage tube was inserted which had to be removed every morning and all thoroughly cleansed with peroxide of hydrogen, an operation which was as hard on me as the child. The inside of the vertebra began to decay and a number of pieces of bone worked out. Other abscesses formed until he had five openings in the back and one in the groin. Sometimes it would be months that he could not walk. Finally his blood was so full of poison that he had a chill every other day. Then in desperation I overcame my prejudices and went to consult Dr. Foo. When he diagnosed his case by just feeling his pulse, I was perfectly astonished. I put him under his care the following week, and today he is perfectly well. I am satisfied that if he had been treated by Dr. Foo at the first that it would have saved him years of suffering, and that his back would not be deformed.

Dr. Foo's treatment is so mild. All he used was poultices, plasters and liniments and the herb teas.

I have found Dr. Foo very reliable in all his dealings. I make this statement in hopes that many subjects of suffering humanity may be cured by Dr. Foo's treatment.

Facts speak for themselves, and if any person is skeptical as to the truth of this statement, they can call on or address,

MRS. A. A. BURCHAM,
San Bernardino, Cal.

A DISLOCATED SHOULDER.

To the Public:

Feeling deeply grateful to Dr. T. Foo Yuen for what he has done for me, I wish to say a few words in his behalf.

Four months ago I had the misfortune to dislocate my right arm at the shoulder. The American doctors set it for me, but it seemed to be very stiff, so I called on Dr. Foo Yuen, who gave me a thorough examination and informed me that he could cure me in a short time. I concluded to try his treatment, and in six days I could use it as well as ever, and in four weeks it was entirely well.

I consider the herb remedies the best for all diseases.

MRS. EMMA FLOOD,
301 East Fifth street, Los Angeles, Cal.

INJURIES TO BONES CURED.

247 East Tenth street,
RIVERSIDE, Cal., August 30, 1896.

Dear Sir:

It is now nearly four years ago since I met with a serious accident, resulting in breaking two ankle bones. I unfortunately fell off the roof of a house I was painting. Local doctors treated me at once, but after a time we found blood congealed under the feet, paralyzing the muscles, which contracted the foot, causing great pain, and crippling me entirely. Some people advised me to undergo an operation, but I strongly objected to such a proceeding. I ultimately heard of Dr. Foo and the remarkable cures he had effected, and determined to try his treatment, which decision I look upon as saving me from being a cripple. The doctor found my system in a very weak and nervous condition; but after a few days' treatment I could rest better, and began to feel an improvement. After three months' treatment I was cured.

In reply to your inquiry as to my present state of health, I am very pleased to say that my general state of health was never better, and my ankles and feet do not trouble me in the least.

I am, yours very truly, W. G. COX.

THREATENED WITH THE LOSS OF A LEG, BUT CURED.

I came to California last October from the East in perfect health, but about the first week in November I sprained my right ankle. I caught cold in it and it inflamed badly. I went to a private hospital for treatment and remained five weeks undergoing treatment and suffering most excruciating pains. I then was advised by the attending physicians to have my leg cut off. I thought my case was not understood by them, and I left the hospital. At this time I had five bad wounds in my leg, and could not put my foot to the ground, and had to walk on crutches with the greatest difficulty. I had a friend who was taking treatment from Dr. T. Foo Yuen. My friend was an Eastern lady, afflicted with asthma, diabetes and other complicated diseases. She had been treated by the best specialists in the East without much relief, but after taking Dr. Foo's remedies she began to improve right along. She brought me one of Dr. Foo's pamphlets, giving an account of little Clara Humphrey's case, which I read with great interest, but was very skeptical about Chinese doctors, and did not pay much attention to it at the time. Later, however, upon inquiry and investigation, I found that Clara Humphrey was perfectly cured. One day my friend asked me to go to Dr. Foo's office for her medicines and requested me to let Dr. Foo feel my pulse and diagnose my case. I did so and was satisfied he knew what he was about, and I concluded to take his remedies at once.

He assured me that he could cure my leg by July; it was then the middle of April. So he gave me medicines, and in July my leg was perfectly cured.

Yours very truly, PROF. F. H. VOLLERY.

BAFFLED THE BEST DOCTORS.

A case in which we recently took much interest and successfully treated was that of Miss Williamson, of Spokane, Washington. That the result was very satisfactory to the patient and to her friends is shown by the following short but decidedly appreciative letter:

SPOKANE, Washington, April 28, 1899.

T. Foo Yuen, Los Angeles, Cal.:

Dear Sir: Just a note to express my gratitude to you for curing my sister of a disease that baffled the best doctors in the West.

I am, yours in gratitude, A. S. WILLIAMSON,

840 Nettie Avenue, Spokane, Wash.

The above case was one of a bone injury to the wrist. This was of long standing, had involved four surgical operations and resulted in blood poisoning. When Miss Williamson commenced treatment with us she was being urged to have the arm amputated, a calamity from which our remedies saved her.

CHAPTER XII.

DISEASES OF THE EYE.

Diseases of the eye are very prevalent. And the indications are that they are constantly increasing in number. This is shown by the great number of people, old and young, who are compelled to wear spectacles, many of them from their earliest school days. It is apparent that there are tendencies at work which are increasing the number of cases of eye difficulty. A number of names are given to the principal diseases of the eye which have no meaning for the average citizen. It is not our purpose to name these disorders, but we do propose to show how some of the most common originate and how they may be successfully treated by the herbal system of medication.

The eye is a very important member of the human body. Nothing is a greater misfortune than loss of sight. It is often worse than death itself. Moreover, from the very delicate and complicated construction of the eye, any disease of this organ is more troublesome and more to be dreaded than disease of almost any other organ. There are many different causes of such diseases. Many of these are remote and unsuspected but nevertheless very frequent. For instance, there is a relation and a bodily connection between the liver and the eye. Any disease of the liver, such as jaundice, for example, immediately shows itself in the eye. Sometimes a person takes a cold which settles in the liver. This, after a little, reaches the eye. Improper diet or the use of unwholesome liquids causes impurities in the stomach and bowels. These impurities are carried through the circulation to the eye and produce cataracts.

Many cases of eye troubles follow other diseases. Thus fevers frequently cause diseases of the eye. Physicians do not have the proper remedies to drive the poison caused by fevers out of the system. They use mineral remedies only and these condense the poison, instead of causing it to expand and scatter and to be thrown out of the body through the skin and other excretory organs. Consequently, the poison settles in the vital organs and from them it sometimes rushes to the brain and produces inflammation of the eye. Sometimes when men are working in the heat of the sun the eyes become affected. Measles and similar diseases, such as eczema, hives and erysipelas, leave poisons in the system when no proper remedies —like the herbal remedies—are used to drive them out. A remnant of poison is left, attacks the vital organs, and finally finds its way to the eyes.

Excessive sexual indulgence puts out the fire of the eye and makes it dark and dull. There is no light in it. Too severe brain labor weakens the eyes. Sometimes there are epidemics in the atmosphere which cause diseases of the eye. These make the eyes red through inflammation and these difficulties usually spread from one member of a family to another until all have been affected. Sometimes a mother who has a disorder of the eye gives it to her child through nursing it. And sometimes children inherit weakness or disease of the eyes from their father or mother, or from both, the trouble descending to them before birth.

We cannot go into all of the details of these difficulties in a brief space, but, in a general way, we may say that our company has treated successfully many cases of these diseases. We have a certain powder which we use in all cases of inflammation of the eye which takes away the pain and at once makes the eye feel cool and comfortable. The patient at once feels easier and correspondingly happy. We also have liquids to use as washes and several different preparations in the shape of fragrant powders which are unequaled in their prompt and pleasant effects.

In connection with these external applications we employ internal remedies which remove the root of the disease. After a cure is once accomplished there will be no further trouble. If we were to use only the external applications to effect temporary relief, and were to neglect the proper internal medication, then the treatment would be worthless in the end. It is necessary to use the external remedies to remove the pain and inflammation and also to employ the internal remedies in order to get at the root and cause of the trouble so that it may not occur again. In this way we accomplish a definite and satisfactory result. Our treatment has saved many people the necessity of wearing glasses all of their lives or of having difficult surgical operations performed. In hundreds of these cases it is unnecessary to use the knife, even to remove cataracts. If the poison which causes the cataract is absorbed and carried away through the circulation and out of the body the cataract will be cured at once. We have remedies which will accomplish this result. It may not appear to be quite as quick as the use of the knife, but it is much more certain and there is much less likelihood of a return of the difficulty.

Many people who have used spectacles for a long time have come to us after exhausting other methods of treatment in an effort to get rid of the spectacles. We have cured many such cases and, after a course of treatment with us, they have cast their spectacles aside never to use them again. The eye is composed of delicate membranes and coatings and it is very natural that these should be quickly affected by disorders of the blood. But it is just as reasonable that when the blood is made pure and the circulation is strong, these disorders should be removed. Any one can understand the philosophy of this, which is simply common sense.

The action of the herbal remedies, which is always soothing, healing and delicate, is much more certain in all diseases of the eye than the harsher action of minerals, or the rude and doubtful expedient of surgical operations. In these diseases, as in all others, nature accomplished wonders with a little assistance in the way of removing those obstructions to the circulation and those unnatural elements in the blood which are products of unnatural ways of life or habits of body. If nature is once set right she can be depended upon to do the rest.

In these diseases, as in all others, the results of experience are the best guide. And our experience in many cases has been very satisfactory. It will be impossible for us to give all the testimonials which we have received from patrons whom we have cured of disorders of the eye. But we shall state a few of the briefest in corroboration of what we have said upon this subject.

A SPEEDY CURE.

WEST PALMDALE, Los Angeles Co., Cal., Oct. 20, 1898.

On the 22d of September, 1898, I was thrown from my road-cart and badly shook up and jarred inside of my head, causing blood to flow from my left ear, nose and mouth. Was also bruised and cut in several places on the face and head, and in particular a bad cut above and below my right eye, causing it to swell shut. The lower half of the eyeball was also badly bruised, causing the blood to settle in it, or, badly blood-shot.

Being under treatment by Dr. T. Foo Yuen before the accident happened, for a complication of diseases, and a general weak and run-down condition, I at once came to his office for treatment of my injuries.

Though still under his treatment, and far from being entirely well, I consider my recovery so far very satisfactory. And in particular think I am very fortunate in regard to my eye, for the cut is pretty well healed.

He put plasters over the cuts to draw out the inflammation, and as soon as the swelling went away so that he could open the eye, he put some kind of cooling medicine on it, and now the blood and inflammation are all gone. In fact the eye is as good as it ever was, except a little scar on the outside of the skin.

Yours respectfully, W. COATES.

VALUABLE EYESIGHT SAVED.

SAN BERNARDINO, Cal., Sept. 18, 1898.

To Whom It May Benefit:

I am forty-three years of age, the last twenty-three of which I have done more or less book-keeping, and some of it under conditions that were very trying to the eyes. About nine years ago while doing a great deal of writing, much of it by lamp light, I first became aware that my eyesight was beoming impaired. The failure at first was so gradual as to occasion but little alarm, and I fully believed that with change of occupation my eyes would soon recover their accustomed strength and clearness of vision. After a time I was enabled to discontinue work by lamp-light, but never succeeded in freeing myself entirely from more or less writing. As a consequence my eyes continued to fail until a point was reached where I could not write or read for more than an hour at a time without suffering much pain and irritation. And if necessity compelled me to continue beyond this point they would blur until the letters would run together, or multiply to such an alarming extent that I would be obliged to desist from further effort. About this time I consulted an optician who finally induced me to wear glasses, and fitted my eyes with two pair. One pair for writing and the other for general use. I found that the glasses rested my eyes, and enabled me to work longer without intermission, and I had become to look upon them as indispensable when my eyelids began to crack and bleed, and were much inflamed, becoming in a short time so painful as to make speedy relief a necessity, which I found where least expected. Dr. Tom Foo Yuen at the time was prescribing for my youngest son, and one day when consulting with him about the boy, out of curiosity, and without knowing that the eye was within his range of treatment, I asked him if he could do anything for my eyes. After a casual examination, his reply was characteristic of the man, for it consisted of the single word "sure."

My experience of Dr. Foo's skill, and confidence in his judgment was such, that while his reply was somewhat of a surprise, I had no hesitancy about submitting my eyes to his treatment, the wisdom of which has been proved by the fact that today my sight is fully restored, all inflammation is gone, and my vision is as clear as it ever has been, as far back as I can remember. I have no need for glasses and do not wear them in-doors or out. The treatment I received was neither painful, disagreeable, or inconvenient to any noticeable degree, and offered relief from the start; and to any who are similarly afflicted I feel perfectly safe in saying, that in Dr. Tom Foo Yuen you will find a competent and skillful physician, fully qualified to carry to a successful issue anything he undertakes, who is safe, sure and humane in all his treatments, and withal—a gentleman in the fullest sense of the word.

I speak advisedly as well as positively in his behalf, for I know him and his work well, and deserving of all praise.

Box 1003, San Bernardino, Cal.   T. G. KELTY.

WAS SPARED A PAINFUL OPERATION.

The Foo and Wing Herb Company, Los Angeles:

Gentlemen: I desire to express my gratitude to you, and praise for your superior system of medicine, both in my own case and that of my son Robert, whom you cured in 1897 of a very severe case of bone injury, called by some doctors "bone cancer." He had been on crutches for three and one-half years and we had in the meantime tried various remedies but found no relief until we went to you. I am pleased to say that through your skillful management and your powerful herbal remedies, my boy was restored to health, and his limb completely healed. I was then thoroughly convinced of the efficacy of your system, and decided at once to try your remedies myself. Mine was an obstinate case of granulated sore eyes. I had tried remedies of various kinds, and treated with several doctors without getting any relief. Was advised by one—as the only relief—to have an operation performed, but I am glad to say that I did not submit, but was spared that severe treatment. I consider myself exceedingly fortunate that I learned of the Chinese system of medicine, and in a few months under your treatment my sight was fully restored, and without taking the chances of losing it altogether by the use of the knife.

I regard the Oriental system of medicine as being superior to all others, especially when administered by the hands of such skillful and scientific doctors as the Foo and Wing Herb Co.

Yours truly, ALBERT A. DEXTER.
San Bernardino, Cal., 1898.

CURED OF A CATARACT IN THE EYE.

The following is from a lady who is thoroughly familiar with our system of treatment, having been cured in 1895 of hemorrhoids and catarrh. Miss McPherson says:

T. Foo Yuen, Los Angeles, Cal.:

Dear Sir: I desire herein to express my kind appreciation of your most skillful treatment in curing my eye of a cataract which was very painful, and for which your treatment was most effectual and complete.

The cataract was so far advanced when I came to you that it affected the sight and had even caused the eyelids to droop somewhat. It was so far advanced that you said to me that I was fortunate that I had not delayed longer in coming to you, and that if I had not come soon you would not have been able to cure me.

My eye is as perfect today as if I had never been troubled with the cataract at all.

While the pain resulting from the application of the remedies to the eye is very severe, lasting from ten to twenty minutes, yet as soon as these moments are passed, the eye feels natural and immediately becomes clear.

I make this acknowledgement that you may know that I fully appreciate your skillful treatment and faithful attention in restoring my eye to its normal condition.

Yours very truly, SADIE J. McPHERSON.

THE CURSE OF HABIT.

We may say, in explanation, that this article is reprinted from a recent issue of the Los Angeles Times. We omit part of the heading that appeared in that paper. The article is as follows:

THE PHILOSOPHY OF THE LIQUOR HABIT FULLY CONSIDERED. ITS CAUSES AND CURE ANALYZED—AN ORIGINAL DESCRIPTION OF THE EVILS OF DRINK.

HOW FRIENDS AND ACQUAINTANCES MAY HELP THE UNFORTUNATE.

Not all of the sermons on intemperance are preached from the pulpit. The columns of the daily papers contain little sermons on this topic every day. "Dead from Alcoholism," "Killed His Wife in a Drunken Rage," "Drunk and Disorderly, Ten Days in Jail," these are some of the headings to the items which constantly remind us that fellow-citizens of ours are on the downward path.

Apart from these extreme cases there are many men who are tired of drink. Alcohol dulls the brain; hinders a man in business; weakens him in the long run, in every way; is a constant drain upon his pocket. Many a man who has been the rounds day after day, night after night, for years, gets tired of the same old course of folly and dissipation. Secretly he would like to stop drinking. But how to do it is the rub. The chains of appetite are upon him. His nervous system imperiously demands the long accustomed stimulants. There are objections to every method of relief offered him. One is too open—excites too much attention and comment. Another is too violent —causes vomiting and purging and all manner of deathly sickness. In others he has no confidence whatever, because he does not believe that they will cure.

WHAT IS HE GOING TO DO ABOUT IT?

There is a cure offered right here in Los Angeles that avoids all of these objections. It is secret, mild and reliable. It has been thoroughly tested. It is not a single drug or preparation made to fit every case, but is a scientific and philosophical system which may be adapted to the varying circumstances of different cases and of all cases. It is in line with other remedies that have perfected hundreds of remarkable cures in other diseases. It employs no poisonous drugs whatever. It is offered by the Foo and Wing Herb Company, of 903 South Olive street, Los Angeles. Those who know this company best will tell you that they always perform whatever they promise to do.

T. FOO YUEN'S ANALYSIS OF THE DRINK HABIT.

In a recent interview Dr. Foo explained his opinions on the use and effects of alcohol, from the standpoint of the physician. Dr. Foo is not an extremist. He has seen enough of the frailties and misfortunes of mankind to make him charitable toward human imperfections. His analysis of the drink habit is interesting because it is based exclusively upon his own observations and physiological investigations. Speaking in his remarkably correct, although sometimes quaint English, Dr. Foo recently spoke on this subject substantially as follows:

"The liquor power goes through the body quicker than anything else in the nature of food or drink. It makes the people strong immediately. Sometimes this is a very good thing. Then why does it finally injure the people? I will try to expain that principle. Anything in food or liquor that is used to strengthen the people must be gentle in its action so that it will help the natural power of the vital organs. But the liquor power goes too quickly and too strong. It is the opposite of the natural power in this respect. Therefore it injures the natural power. So, if the people use liquor for a long time then the natural power of the body loses its gentle effect and then it waits for the coming of the liquor power. And when the man has taken the liquor he feels strong. If there is no liquor taken then the man feels weak, because he has created a desire by using liquor for a long time and the desire has created a habit.

HOW THE LIQUOR HABIT HURTS.

"The strength of the liquor goes through the body so quickly that it carries the gastric juices with it. It not only rushes through the body, but it goes out again through the pores of the skin. But there is only a small amount of the gastric juices and if a great deal of this is wasted through the pores of the body then there is not enough left in the stomach for the processes of digestion. Then the stomach gets dry and does not furnish enough saliva to the mouth. And there comes a great thirst. The man wants to drink all of the time. He drinks too much whiskey and too much water. The stomach is constantly flooded and the constant deluge of cold drinks creates the first injury.

"Again, the liquor power is of the fire element. It makes the body warm very quickly and if too much liquor is taken it causes an inflammation. This is the second injury. And both of these injurious effects, the dampness and the inflammation, work together and there is malarial poisoning which may become very bad. This is irrespective of climate. It is as likely to occur in a good climate as in a bad climate.

HOW WHISKEY HURTS THE BLOOD AND THE BRAIN.

"Also, there is in the blood of man a little substance which the American doctor calls a corpuscle. And when the man has had the liquor habit a long time then the corpuscles in his blood become used to the habit also. Then, when he begins to see that he has made a mistake, that he is injuring his business, or has trouble with his family, he wants to try to stop the habit, but the corpuscle does not like to stop the habit. It has a desire all the time for the liquor and the man cannot control himself. He is not independent.

"Again the principle of the liquor is of the fire element and its power rushes. So, when a man has taken a drink of whiskey the effect goes up to the brain at once. And the brain all the time has the liquor power to help the brain. Then the brain feels strong. But when the power of the liquor is gone then the man feels weaker than before. Also, the strength of the liquor holds the brain power very hard. Then the brain cannot perform its natural functions, and all the time the liquor power controls the brain; the brain cannot control anything. Then the man becomes dull and drunk. His mind is not clear. And so his nature is all changed. The good nature becomes bad. But we cannot tell all of the injuries from liquor. There are many other ways of injury. We prepare remedies to stop this habit in more than one way. If the man himself desires to stop; if he understands that he has made a mistake and has made up his mind to stop, then we will try to clean out his system first and afterwards to stop the habit. This is one way. But other people do not want to stop the habit. Still, sometimes the parents like to stop the habit in the children, or the sister in the brother, or the wife in the husband. For these cases we have another kind of medicine which may be put into the food or drink of the man. He will not know about it. But after he has taken this his appetite will be removed. This is another very excellent way. In all of these cases it is necessary to change the old blood for new blood and so to change the desire and the appetite. We must help the natural powers of the body to overcome the power of the liquor. And this is the only way in which the man can be permanently cured."

A CORRECT DIAGNOSIS.

We submit that the above is a correct diagnosis, that it contains in a nutshell the whole philosophy of the drink habit and its cure. No long-winded dissertation, full of big words and technical terms, could be clearer or more complete. We may summarize briefly the advantages of Dr. Foo's treatment, as follows:

(1.) It is absolutely secret. None of your friends need know that you are under treatment for the liquor habit. They will not suspect it except as they notice it in your improved appearance and clearer expression of ideas.

(2.) It is perfectly harmless. The treatment is adapted to your bodily strength and condition. All of the medicinal agents employed are absolutely innocent and non-poisonous. Many of the liquor cures upon the market produce very injurious effects. None of these can possibly occur from this cure. The patient is strengthened and assisted in every way. He becomes a man again in the full sense of the term, with strong nerves, a sound digestion, a clear brain and a normal performance of all the vital functions.

(3.) This company has remedies that may be administered without the patient's knowledge or consent. These are powerful, but harmless. They are an antidote to the liquor habit. They take away the desire for liquors—not all at once but by degrees. They take the place of the whiskey stimulus and as the desire grows less the man does not feel weak and nerveless, but stronger and better. He begins to see that he can do without the whiskey. In many cases the taste and smell of whiskey become actually repulsive. From this point a cure is easy.

(4.) The processes of this cure are slow and permanent, not violent and transitory as is the case with so many alleged cures. There are none of the painful and ditressing vomitings and purgings resulting from some of these, none of the lasting injuries resulting from others. The healing effects extend through the whole body, through the blood and the brain and all of the nerves and tissues. Little by little these are cleansed and renewed. They are nourished and sustained. When the process is complete the man is literally made over and the baneful desire is gone, along with the vitiated blood and tissues which were the seat of that desire. Could any cure be more complete or satisfactory?

(5.) These cures are worth the money paid for them. They are not offered for a dollar or two—no cures worthy the name can be sold for such a ridiculous price. But many people have paid for high-priced cures two, three, four and even a greater number of times. They were not permanent. They may have removed the desire for liquors temporarily, but they did not give the patient the necessary assistance to carry him along and to prevent him from slipping back into the embraces of his old habit. Therefore, in the end they were very expensive. But the man who takes remedies of the Foo and Wing Herb Company need never touch liquor again. If he does there is absolutely no excuse for him.

A SINGLE TESTIMONIAL.

The Foo and Wing Herb Company has made many cures of the liquor habit, and also of the morphine and other drug habits. But persons cured of these are naturally very much averse to the publication of their names. For this reason this company has no extensive testimonials to offer along this line. But the following references may be given in regard to one case which is typical of numerous others:

LOS ANGELES, Cal., November 25, 1898.

To Whom It May Concern:

We, the undersigned, can testify to the merits of the liquor cure for sale by the Foo and Wing Herb Company, from a case which came under our personal observation.

Some six weeks ago a gentleman in this city was given this cure without his knowledge. It was administered by his wife.

He had been using intoxicants all his life, and had reached a point where the habit had taken a very serious hold on him. He had taken the Keeley cure twice, and had lost his position through his habits of intoxication, and was a source of great anxiety to his friends.

The remedy worked like a charm in this case. In about three or four weeks the young man lost all appetite for liquor, gained in flesh and strength, and seemed completely restored to health.

It was a wonderful change and surprise to all his friends and acquaintances.

MRS. N. IDELLA VESPER,
584 Summit avenue, Pasadena, Cal.
MRS. E. R. BRITTEN,
711 Court street, Los Angeles.
GEORGE W. HAZARD,
1307 S. Alvarado street, Los Angeles.

NO CASES TOO SEVERE.

This imperial remedy brings all degrees of the liquor habit under control. It has snatched victims from the very clutches of delirium tremens. It soon relieves the nervous tension which is the principal cause and the most distressing symptom of mania from liquor habit. Then it gradually places the patient upon his feet as already described. This is a most important point to consider, for many unfortunates addicted to liquor will refuse all proffered assistance until the intense suffering of approaching mania compels them to submit. Every drinking man who feels and knows that his habit is getting beyond his control should pause and consider whether he is willing to go farther and until he finds himself in danger of the mad-house.

A CHANCE FOR PHILANTHROPISTS.

In this remedy temperance reformers may find a practical use for their energies. Here is something definite to offer a man who is the slave of habit, or a wife who is silently suffering untold misery from day to day as she watches her husband going deeper and deeper in his pitiful degradation. Given a sufficient motive to undertake a cure, on the part either of the sufferer or of his friends, there is no excuse for not employing these remedies. Everybody knows of such cases as these, and very often a word fitly spoken at the right time may lead to the reformation of a man worth saving, and to bringing happiness into the abode of wretchedness and despair.

HOW TO SECURE THESE REMEDIES.

There is only one way to secure these remedies. They are sold in only one place in the United States, and that is the office of the Foo and Wing Herb Company, at 903 South Olive street, Los Angeles. They may, however, be sent by mail or express to any point. It is not necessary that the doctors should actually see the patient. But they require a clear statement of the case rendered, either in person or by letter. Then the remedies will be furnished in accordance with the circumstances of each case. When convenient, a personal interview is undoubtedly the best. But it is not, strictly speaking, necessary. Write to the doctors or call upon them, as is the most convenient. In either case you will receive careful attention and every consideration.

SUBSTANTIAL TOKENS OF APPRECIATION.

It will doubtless occur to many readers of this book that the prices for our remedies for home treatment are higher than the prices asked for the patent medicines sold in the American drug stores. This is true if you consider the question of price alone. But when you consider the question of price as compared with the benefits received the prices of our remedies are not too high. In fact, many of our patrons, the persons best able to judge because most familiar with what our remedies accomplish, have said to us that they consider our prices very reasonable indeed. When health is at stake that remedy is cheapest which restores health. A remedy which accomplishes no good is dear even if given for nothing. A remedy which cures is worth almost any price. When you consider this question from this point of view you will see that our remedies are simply invaluable.

It has been a very common occurrence for patrons of T. Foo Yuen to express their pleasure with his methods and with the results accomplished in a very substantial manner, a fact which is a sufficient proof that he has not placed too high a valuation upon his remedies. Not only have many of his patrons paid full prices for their treatment but they have become and have remained steadfast friends and have given him, from time to time, expensive presents as tokens of their personal esteem. We think it proper to mention a few of the most important of these as illustrating the points herein discussed. Of the smaller presents, which have been innumerable, we shall make no mention, not speaking of any worth less than fifty dollars each.

For instance, he was very much pleased recently at receiving a handsome cut-glass punch bowl and mirror from a recent patient, Capt. A. Bassett of Sioux City, Iowa, accompanied by the following appreciative letter, the bowl having been forwarded from San Francisco, at which city Capt. Bassett had stopped on his way East.

San Francisco, Cal., March 17, 1899.

Dr. T. Foo Yuen, 903 S. Olive St., Los Angeles, Cal.:

Dear Sir:—I send today, by express, a cut-glass punch bowl and mirror, which please accept as a slight token of my esteem and gratitude for the skill and care of which I have been the recipient under your treatment, which have resulted in such a vast improvement in my health.

Wishing you a long life and much happiness, I remain,

Yours very respectfully, A. BASSETT,

1723 Ross St., Sioux City, Iowa.

The value of this handsome gift is not less than one hundred and fifty dollars, but, like all the others herein mentioned, it is appreciated by Dr. Foo, not for its money cost, but for the fact that it comes from a friend and is a testimonial to the fact that, by his skill as a physician, he has been able to accomplish a noteworthy good to a friend. In the same spirit we may mention the following.

A diamond studded gold watch, from Mrs. Gertrude E. Samo of 1818 E. Second street, Los Angeles, value $250; an iron safe from J. H. Britton, agent for the Mosler Safe Co., of 334 and 336 N. Main street, Los Angeles, value $125; an oil painting of Dr. Foo from the well-known artist, William G. Cogswell of 1138 S. Flower street. This was a New Year's gift, on the first of January, 1898. Its value is $250. Captain C. Taylor of 520 S. Grand avenue, presented Dr. Foo with a thirty-day clock, which hangs in his office, price $125. S. R. Crowe of Redlands gave him a handsome buffalo-horn chair, worth $125. Mrs. W. J. Anderson of Chicago remembered the doctor with a diamond ring valued at $100. Mrs. Cox of Riverside sent him the deed to a lot in Riverside. Mrs. Hall sent a beautiful picture valued at $50, and there have been many others.

Among these remembrances which Dr. Foo values most high are two from Mrs. Katharine Ellis, who is Mrs. Samo's mother. In 1896, Mrs. Ellis, then 82 years of age, was treated by Dr. Foo for eye troubles so successfully that her sight was better than for many year previous to that time. To show her appreciation of this fact she embroidered a handsome sofa pillow, with an elaborate design in seven different colors, and presented it to him, as a present for New Year's, 1897. Early in the present year Mrs. Ellis took a severe cold which Dr. Foo cured. She then embroidered an afghan for his office chair, being at this time 84 years of age.

The writer submits that these tokens of good will indicate that there is a greater benefit to be derived from these remedies than the price would indicate. But this is a matter which each person can very readily test for himself. A few doses of the remedies will cost but little—say of those for the cure of colds, for example. But they will save many times their cost in the price of doctor's visits. Those, if any there are, who are not satisfied with the results of this test need not try again. But we believe that it will be found to be true that those who will use these remedies faithfully and as directed, and with the idea of checking disease at the outset and not waiting until it has become deeply seated in the system, will find that their expenses for doctors' bills and medicines will be reduced to one-half, every year, and that the trouble, anxiety and suffering from disease will be reduced in the same proportion.

Remember, in a word, that it is not what a thing costs but what it does which determines its value. A remedy at a dollar a dose which saves life is better than a remedy at one cent a dose which does no good whatever and simply leads a patient on with delusive hopes until his condition becomes incurable by any means whatever. This is too often the result of cheap medication.

(The following article is reprinted substantially as it appeared in the Los Angeles Times for New Year's, 1902.)

APPENDICITIS.

A Growing Fad of Modern Surgery — A Quick and Certain Method of Demise — A New Name for an Ancient Foe of the Human Race—Some Suggestions for Those who Fear this Prevalent and Fatal Malady.

That little, curly attachment at the inner extremity of the large intestines in the human body, which looks, in the pictures of the human anatomy, like the dried-up stem of a melon or a pumpkin, is giving people no end of trouble nowadays. Every week somebody dies of appendicitis, the name assigned by our modern doctors to whatever form of inflammation interferes with the functions of this apparently trifling, but really important, portion of our bodies. The surgeon's knife is supposed to be the only cure and this, in most cases, is not a cure, for it means a shock to the system that results in death. Everyone has lost friends by this disease and thousands live in nameless terror lest it attack them also.

SOME EXCEPTIONS TO THE RULE.

Although the knife is usually considered the only way of getting rid of appendicitis—in spite of the difficult and dangerous operation involved—yet there are American physicians who will not resort to this extreme measure and emphatically assert that they have cured numerous cases of appendicitis without surgery. That this is entirely possible is proved by the results secured by the Oriental doctors in this country, who never resort to surgery. Yet they often cure appendicitis, even in an advanced stage. What is more, they have a consistent and reasonable theory of the uses of this little vermiform appendix in the human body.

Mr. W. A. Hallowell Jr., a resident of this city, became interested in this subject through a personal experience of the painful sort that many surgeons have undergone. Some months ago a brother, E. A. Hallowell, formerly mayor of Belleville, Kansas, afterwards a resident of Kansas City, commenced to experience the painful symptoms that foreshadow appendicitis. He consulted different physicians, but received no relief. His brother advised him to come to this city and try the Oriental remedies and sent him testimonials of cures accomplished by them. He was very favorably impressed by the testimonials, but his business affairs would not permit him to leave Kansas City. He finally submitted to an operation, with the usual result, death.

FOUND A BETTER WAY.

It seemed to the surviving Mr. Hallowell, the one residing in this city, that there ought to be some remedy which, at least when taken in good time, might avert disaster of this sort. He therefore asked T. Foo Yuen, the president of the Foo and Wing Herb Company, and the most noted Oriental physician in America, to explain to him his ideas of the function of the vermiform appendix and his theories of that fatal disorder, appendicitis. The information which he received upon this subject was as follows:

"As you will see from the picture the vermiform appendix is attached, like the stem of a melon, to one extremity of the large intestine. It is a continuation of the cord which runs the whole length of the intestine and is everywhere attached to the large intestine by little muscles. The Chinese call this an auxiliary intestine. From its position it is so closely related to the large intestine that whenever the one is affected by any disease the other is affected also. The appendix has a small opening into its upper extremity, but none from its lower extremity. Therefore, small substances, under certain conditions, may enter it but are very difficult to dislodge.

FUNCTIONS OF THE VERMIFORM APPENDIX.

"Now, after the digested food passes from the stomach the lighter portions go into the small intestines and parts are assimilated into the blood and the heavier portions go into the large intestine, as refuse, and finally pass away from the body. The appendix has an expansive and contractile power and assists in this separation of the digestible portions of the food from that which is merely refuse. That which goes into the small intestines is very light, but that which goes into the large intestine is coarse and heavy. When the separation takes place the appendix expands and furnishes the power to the large intestine to receive these coarser elements of the food and to hold them until they are discharged in the natural way. Whenever the appendix is affected by disease and loses its power to assist the large intestine this function is imperfectly performed and trouble results.

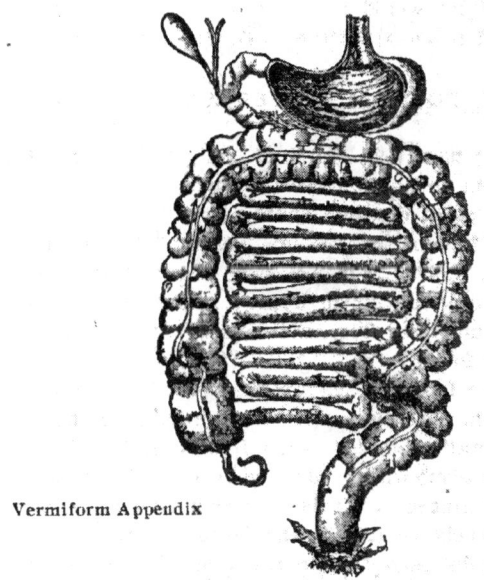

Vermiform Appendix

THREE PRINCIPAL FORMS OF APPENDICITIS.

"When the appendix becomes affected the resulting disorder manifests itself in one of three principal phases of symptoms. The first set of complications arises when improper food is eaten or food which is difficult of digestion. Then portions of this undigested food remain too long in the intestines and cause inflammation in the large intestine. This passes to the smaller intestines, the natural juices which assist in the important functions of this portion of our bodies are dried up, the bowels do not act properly and poisons are engendered by the failure to rid the body, in time, of the mass of undigested food and refuse. Some of this poison finds its way into the appendix, which loses its power to assist the large intestine and it has, also, no power to throw off the poisons already received. Therefore it becomes swollen, inflamed and painful. This was the condition in which Mr. L. F. Holtz was when he came to us and commenced to take our remedies. I will show you his testimonial.

"Another form is not always caused by improper food but may be due to taking cold or to a catarrhal condition of the system or to any poison which exists in the body. The mucus of catarrh or any other poison in the system may find its way into the large intestine and from that into the appendix, which is like a very small tube closed at its lower extremity, and therefore it is very hard to remove the poison that has once entered. This soon sets up an inflammation and causes pain, which is very difficult to cure. The pain may not be severe at first, but it gradually increases. Sometimes the poisons thus engendered follow the course of the intestines and cause piles, as in the case of Mrs. Lanning.

"The third form of disorder to the appendix is from a lowering of the natural heat of the body. The Chinese theory is that this natural heat has its origin in the kidneys. Be that as it may be, whenever this heat is sufficient, then the appendix expands and assists, as we have shown, in separating the solid from the liquid materials of the food at the point where the large and small intestines are united. But when there is not sufficient power from the kidneys then the appendix also becomes weak and loses its power to control the separation of the liquid from the solid portions of the food. The appendix itself becomes swollen and inflamed and fails to do its work. The food is not properly separated. There is bloating and distress and pain in the side, rumbling in the bowels and diarrhoea. But the pains are not at the same points as in the other forms of this disease. This condition may exist for a long time before it takes on the virulent form that ends in death. This was the form of disorder from which Mrs. Cowan suffered, whose testimonial I will also show you.

THE SEED-LODGING THEORY.

"It is commonly supposed by our American doctors," said Mr. Hallowell, "that all this trouble is caused by seeds or other foreign substances lodging in the appendix and setting up an inflammation. This is shown, they think, by the fact that such substances are often found in the appendix when an operation is made and the appendix is removed. What have you to say in regard to this?"

"I think that this rarely happens," said T. Foo Yuen, "although it is doubtless true that such substances are sometimes found as you have stated. But this is not so much a cause of the disease as one of its results. When the system is perfectly healthy and all the functions of digestion and nutrition are properly performed nothing can lodge in the appendix. Nature takes care of that. But when this little organ becomes inflamed and swollen it may be opened at its upper extremity enough to permit seeds to lodge there, and if that once happens it is extremely difficult to get them out again and, of course, they are very irritating and make the trouble infinitely worse. So the mistake is made, when these are found, of assuming that they were the cause of the disease. And this condition, as I understand it, is what American physicians mean when they speak of appendicitis. This, I think, is incorrect, for any inflammation which may exist for a long time, is a disease of the little organ involved and might properly be called by this name."

OUGHT TO EDUCATE THE PEOPLE.

"I think," Mr. Hallowell continued, "that you ought to print your ideas on this subject so that the people may understand and may secure relief before it is too late. Now, my brother was ill for a long time before the 30th day of last September, when the operation was performed in his case. A few days later he was dead. All his family were sorry, then, that he had not taken your remedies at first, but of course, it was too late. Undoubtedly the same experience happens often."

"Yes," was the reply, "that is very true. No one ought to delay or trifle with the symptoms of so severe a disorder. I have often tried to discuss these subjects, for the benefit of the public, in my articles in the newspapers and in the books that the Foo and Wing Herb Company has published. Any persons interested may come to the office of this company, at 903 S. Olive street, Los Angeles, and ask any questions that they desire and discuss these matters with us. We do everything in our power to assist those who are seeking to regain their health."

THE FIRST PRINCIPLES OF A CURE.

"Can you tell me, in a few words," asked Mr. Hallowell, "something about the way in which your remedies accomplish a cure in such a painful and serious disease?"

"It is very simple," said T. Foo Yuen, "provided you thoroughly understand the causes. So great a disturbance to the system is quickly manifest in the pulse, and our pulse diagnosis tells us at once how far the trouble has progressed. Then our herbal remedies, which contain no poisons, act very gently yet very effectively. They soon reduce the inflammation and cause the secretion of a new supply of the gastric and intestinal juices upon which the health of the organs in question depends. Then the circulation of the blood in these parts is quickened and the poisons there are removed by absorption and by carrying them off through the natural channels. This cannot all be done at once—a cure in these cases requires a little time, but it is certain if the trouble is taken in time. Of course, there are cases that are absolutely beyond relief, because they have been permitted to go too far. The cure of any disease is simply a question of providing the proper remedy in the right place. We have the remedies that are especially adapted to these disorders and that is the whole secret of a cure. The only danger is in delay."

Following are the

TESTIMONIALS REFERRED TO ABOVE.

The first is from Mr. L. F. Holtz and is as follows:

"I was taken seriously ill last year at my home, Phoenix, British Columbia, and two doctors said it was appendicitis. I went to Spokane, Washington, to consult with doctors at the Sisters' Hospital of that city, who declared that my disease was incurable, but my life might be prolonged a few months by dieting and with good care. I was at the hospital for three weeks and suffered terrible pains in the intestines and right side during that time. From there I went to

Kansas City, Omaha and Chicago, and was under the care of the best physicians in each of those cities, but without obtaining relief. Finally I accidentally heard of some wonderful cures effected by Dr. T. Foo Yuen of the Foo and Wing Herb Company, Los Angeles, and placed myself under his care. After five months' treatment I was thoroughly cured and am now working in the mines at Phoenix, B. C., in perfect health."

(Signed) L. F. HOLTZ.

Mrs. J. C. Lanning of Bloomington, San Bernardino County, California, has sent us a fine testimonial of the results of treatment in her case, which cured her of sciatica, rheumatism, piles, and appendicitis. The testimonial is as follows:

NOTEWORTHY CURE OF MRS. J. C. LANNING.

RIALTO, California, October 25, 1901.

The Foo and Wing Herb Company, Los Angeles, Cal.:

Gentlemen:—As one of those who have been restored to health by the use of your remedies, after a very long and painful illness, I take pleasure in giving you a brief statement of the principal facts in my case.

My illness commenced in my Canadian home some eight years ago, and I finally came to California, in the hope that a change of climate would restore my health. I consulted many physicians and took various form of treatment, both in the East and in California, but without receiving any benefit. The doctors who prescribed for me gave my troubles different names and had numerous theories regarding them, but all of the treatment was equally unsuccessful. Some of the physicians said that I had nervous prostration, an exhaustion of nerve energy. One diagnosed the case as inflammation of the bladder, another as sciatica rheumatism. I had intense neuralgiac and rheumatic pains and was swollen with dropsy. I had taken arsenic until my face was bleached white. I was burning with inward fever, yet my circulation was so poor that I felt cold, even while in mud baths at Arrowhead Springs at a temperature of more than a hundred degrees. I took these baths and tried to sweat away the poisons in my system, but the baths only weakened me, without curing the disease.

I heard of the Foo and Wing Herb Company by accident from Mrs. Motherspaw, a lady living in Highlands, who had been cured of rheumatism by their remedies. Some of the physicians of this company were then making trips, every two weeks, to San Bernardino, near which town I was then residing and still reside. They had just been there and would not come again for two weeks. During that time my husband thought that I was at the point of death and wanted to call an American physician, but I would not consent. I could not go to see the doctor, but he sent remedies to me by my husband. I took them and at once commenced to get better. After the third dose I was able to get up and walk to the door.

The last stage in my treatment was the removal of poisons from my system which had taken the form of a severe case of piles. This was accomplished by remedies prepared by Dr. Foo's brother, Dr.

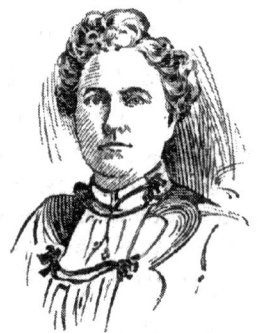

MRS. J. C. LANNING.

Tom Leong. I think that this disease would have taken the form of appendicitis if it had continued. But an ointment, used in the rectum, drew the poisons from the intestines, and the vermiform appendix and removed this danger.

After that I began to gain strength very rapidly. I now appear to be, and feel that I am, as well as anyone, having a degree of health and of pleasure in life such as I had not known for many years.

I am as thoroughly convinced as I am of anything that I should have died within a month if I had not been fortunate enough to hear of the Foo and Wing Herb Company, from a person who had every confidence in them, as a result of her own experience. My own case has given me equal confidence, and I hope that this statement may be of benefit to others by pointing out the way to health. I wish to add to this statement the fact that I have always found T. Foo Yuen and his associates perfect gentlemen in every sense of the word, always considerate and polite in their conduct towards their patients, and men of honor, refinement and dignity.

MRS. J. C. LANNING.

Mrs. Henrietta Cowan, of this city, wife of a physician, had been afflicted for two years with the third form of this disorder as described above. She was cured by our herbal remedies and has written us a very appreciative letter describing her symptoms and the results of her use of the remedies suggested by us. This letter is as follows:

No. 933 Bellevue Avenue,
LOS ANGELES, Cal., Dec. 10, 1901.

To Whom It May Concern:

I wish to make a voluntary statement of my experience of Dr. T. Foo Yuen's treatment in my case, for the benefit of those who may be similarly afflicted. I had been ill with chronic diarrhoea for two years; had to diet all the time, there being only a few kinds of food that I could eat, and I received but little nourishment from anything.

As a consequence my blood was very poor and my system in a run-down and debilitated condition. I had been under treatment from a number of our best physicians with no apparent benefit. There was some temporary relief but it seemed as if I was always taking one step forward and two steps backward until I finally despaired. Having heard about Dr. Foo from a lady whom he had cured, after her case had been pronounced incurable by six of our best physicians, I went to him and without my telling him a word about my ailment, he told me that I had inflammation in the stomach and a catarrhal condition of the system; that I had had malaria for a long time; he described the discomfort under which I constantly labored; the pain and rumbling in the bowels particularly on my right side, and similar symptoms, and described my condition more fully than I could have described it myself. This diagnosis by the pulse fully decided me in favor of taking a test treatment of two weeks. For I thought that a doctor who could tell in that way the exact nature of the disease was certainly the one who would know the best remedies to use in its cure.

Dr. Foo has since told me that my condition was one which frequently leads us to the serious and usually incurable malady known as appendicitis, from which we hear of so many deaths nowadays. Our American doctors do not give it this name until it involves the vermiform appendix and when it reaches that stage it is usually beyond remedy. I was fortunate in checking the trouble before it had gone so far as that for I experienced a benefit from the first dose of Dr. Foo's herbal remedies, and, before the two weeks were up, I had decided to continue. I have now taken the herbs four and a half months, the time set by Dr. Foo, in the first place, as necessary to complete a cure, and have been so greatly improved that I feel like a new creature and find difficulty in fully expressing my gratitude. It certainly gives me great pleasure to add this testimonial to the many which Dr. Foo has received from others of his patrons.

One point which impressed me greatly in favor of the herbal remedies is that they have accomplished a cure with so little disturbance to the system in general. Their action is so gentle, and, at the same time, so searching that I feel as if they have removed my whole body and yet I have been able to do more work while taking them than at any time for two years. I have been asked whether I had to take lizards, toads, bugs, beetles, etc., and I wish to say, in regard to this absurd impression, that these herbs are the cleanest and most daintily prepared remedies I ever saw. It is true that their taste is often bitter and the dose seems large, but a great relief, nevertheless, from the "every hour" or "four times a day" directions of our own doctors.

I suppose that there may be Chinese quack so-called doctors who use bugs and lizards in their alleged prescriptions, but that Dr. Foo would use anything of this sort is simply preposterous. I always found him an amiable, refined and courteous gentleman, charitable and kind to all alike. I wish him long life and prosperity, for his life is, every day, a blessing to the sick.

MRS. HENRIETTA COWAN.

The following letter also bears on this subject:

CURE OF CATARRH AND THREATENED APPENDICITIS.

OLIVE, Orange Co., Cal., Dec. 1, 1901.

The Foo and Wing Herb Company, Los Angeles, Cal.:

Gentlemen: I had been troubled with catarrh for several years, which had reached a stage which, as I am told, often poisons the

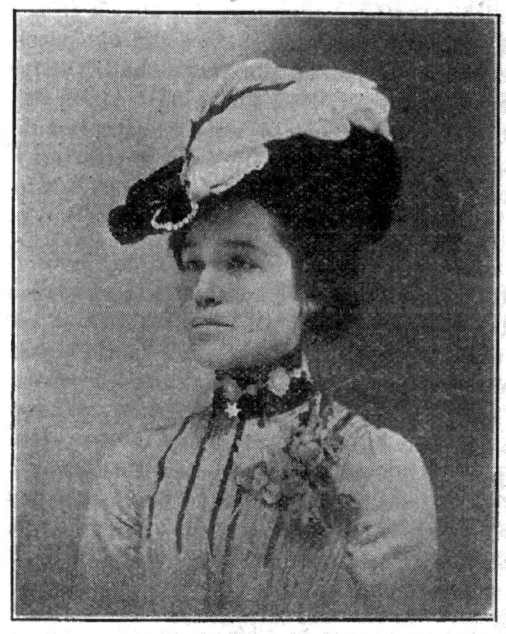

BELLE CARPENTER.

system and leads to appendicitis. After hearing of the cures accomplished by the Foo and Wing Herb Company I decided to go and see them. I was greatly surprised when I received a correct diagnosis of my case by the pulse alone and without the asking of a question. From that time I had a great desire to take the treatment.

I find that these remedies are very searching and purifying to the blood and also invigorating to the whole system. I know personally of many, besides myself, who have received great benefit from them. I believe that these methods of treatment are far superior to those of our own physicians and the remedies are administered in a much gentler manner than our own. There is one great advantage in using these pure herbs, namely, that they do not have the poisoning effect upon the system that many of the minerals administered by our own home physicians have. I can truly say that I believe that T. Foo Yuen, president of this company, has done more for me than any physician I know of could have done and my gratitude to him is unbounded.

I consider him a highly educated gentleman and can gladly recommend him to those needing medical assistance.

Yours truly, BELLE CARPENTER.

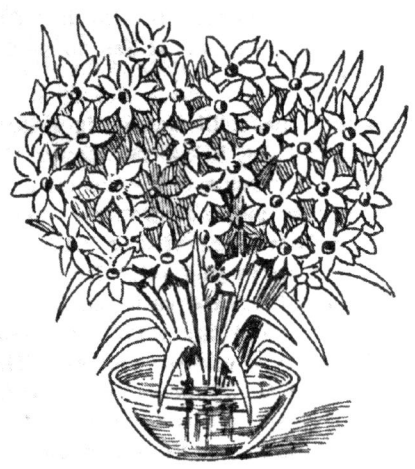

SACRED LILY OF CHINA.

LEGEND OF THE SACRED LILY OF CHINA.

The Symbol of Peace, Good Will and Happiness Among the Chinese—Story of Its Origin—Traditions Allied to the Teachings of Christianity—How Good Deeds Brought Their Reward and Conferred Prosperity Upon a Deserving Family.

The Chinese New Year is the time of universal peace and goodwill among all who owe allegiance to the Flowery Kingdom, whether they are living in their native land or are scattered among foreign peoples. The Sacred Lily of China is a conspicuous feature of all celebrations of this holiday season, of all festivities and of all religious ceremonies. I intend to describe the origin of this wonderful flower. It is a monopoly of the Cum Ying Fong family, of the country of Chong Chow and the state of Foo-chien. Many years ago Cum Ying Fong was only a man's name, but it is now the name of a great and wealthy corporation or company. The Sacred Lily grows in only one place, where it has been growing for the last 500 years. Before that time this flower was never seen. It has no seed, but grows from the atmosphere.

Now the place where these lilies grow is a large piece of very stony ground, which spreads out below the mouth of a canyon in the mountains. When the heavy rains come the muddy water from the mountains spreads over this piece of ground. When the water subsides a thin layer of soil is left, and after a little, nobody knows how or why, the lily bulbs appear in this soil. Here they are allowed to grow for a time, and then they are gathered and sold. Those that are to be used at once are placed in a vessel or vase of water, usually upheld in the dish by a little pile of pebbles. Then, without any nourishment from the ground, but fed entirely by the water and the atmosphere, first the long, green, slender stalks of the plant appear, and in a short time buds follow, then there is a mass of beautiful white and gold lilies with a very sweet and penetrating odor, which, from a single bunch of these lilies will fill a large apartment with fragrance. Frequently these lilies grow to two feet or more, bud and blossom, all within a couple of weeks. The flowers endure a couple of weeks longer and then gradually fade away.

But the bulbs may also be kept a long time and shipped to a great distance by a very simple process. If it is not desired to obtain the flower at once, the bulbs, about the size and something of the shape of an ordinary Bermuda onion, are surrounded with a layer of plastic mud, something like adobe, a sort of clay, which is pressed firmly about the bulbs and covers them completely. This casing of waxlike clay is permitted to dry in the sun, and becomes very hard. The bulb is thus enclosed in an air-tight coating and lies dormant for a long time. This covering of clay is very hard, and the lilies, so protected, are shipped to all parts of China, to America, and to other countries by the hundreds of thousands. When it is desired to grow the flower the covering is broken, little slits or gashes are made in the bulb with a sharp knife, so that the shoots or sprouts may the more easily come into the air. The bulb is placed in water and it soon sends forth its long, thread-like roots downward and the thin, flat, delicate lily leaves upward into the atmosphere. These broad leaves feed voraciously upon the air and the roots rapidly absorb the water. So the quick growth and bloom of the plant are the result.

When the plant is once blossomed its beauty is gone forever. The stalks may be cut away and the bulb may be placed in the ground, where it will grow after a fashion, but it will not flower as before. Neither will it throw off shoots, or new bulbs, from which the lilies may be grown. The mission of the flower has been fulfilled, and its dies forever. Not until the rains of another season send a new supply of the tiny bulbs, which grow nobody knows how, in only one spot in all the world, will the splendid flower again smile upon those who love it. The Chinese have made it the sacred flower of their country, because of this mysterious origin and because of its great beauty and wonderful fragrance. It is a symbol of all life in the mystery of its birth, coming, as it does, from some source which the mind of man cannot fathom, and disappearing forever when it has lived its little, though beautiful, life. For this reason they regard this flower with reverence and a love that others do not appreciate unless they understand the circumstances.

Every year, about September, there is a big rainstorm and then the water from the mountain runs down into the stony ground of the Cum Ying Fong farm. Here this flower originated in a mysterious way, being a present from the God to a good man, and I shall tell you how this came about. Five hundred years ago Cum Fing Fong, a good man, was a citizen of the county of Chong Chow, state of Foochien. When he was very young his father died, and he was very dutiful to his mother. He had an elder brother named Cum Ti Fong. The family was fairly prosperous. Ying Fong did not look very smart, but he was a great student and fond of books, and had more power than common in his mind. He was very glad to see the Chinese "Book of the Good Doctrine," which is like the Bible, and Ying Fong was a good Christian, as his book taught him to be.

After eighteen years his mother died, and the property was divided between Ying Fong and his brother Ti Fong. The brother said that the property should be divided into two parts, and wrote numbers on two pieces of paper, and put them in a tube. Each was to draw a number, which was to tell which half of the property he should have. But the brother wrote the same thing on two papers, each indicating the stony part of the farm. Then he wrote a paper for the good part of the property, and put it up his sleeve. Ying Fong drew a paper from the tube which gave him the stony part, and Ti Fong brought the paper from his sleeve which gave him the good part. But Ying Fong was generous and did not doubt his brother. So he took the stony ground and was happy just the same. But all the good property belonged to the brother by the number which he had.

So Ti Fong became rich, but Ying Fong could not make money from the stony land, and he became poor after that. Then a friend explained to him the trick that his brother had played, and tried to have him cause the brother to be arrested, but Ying Fong said that he would not do so, and said: "I saw my mother when she was living; she allowed him everything, and when my brother would do some little bad thing she loved him still and was very good to him. I want to be of the same heart and mind as my mother." So he let the brother go as before. And when the New Year or any holiday or birthday came he gave his brother many good presents and said that it was good, when his father and mother were dead, to see his brother still living. The natural love he had for his brother was like the love of a child for its mother.

When Ti Fong saw that his brother was so good to him his heart was changed to love him and to give him some money, but his wife, Mrs. Ti Fong, stopped him and said: "Your brother, Ying Yong, is ignorant and he has no mind for earning money. You cannot tell him how to earn money, but let him try to earn money all the time. His family is too big. You can help him a short time, you cannot help him all the time." So the woman, by her smart tongue, changed her husband's mind, and he did not try to help his brother.

But Ying Fong worked for other men and was very honest. Everybody liked him and paid him higher wages than common, and when he earned money he tried to help the poor and the sick people all the time. He had married when twenty years old a good wife, good natured, very kind and as good as he was. And ten years after his marriage, one September, he took cold. And he had a high fever and could not work.

And after the sickness was better he was lame so long that he could not make money, and the food was all gone, because he had all the time tried to help the poor people and had not tried to keep his money. He had three children, two sons and a girl, who were crying from hunger. His wife tried to cook sweet potatoes for the children, and he and his wife ate very little and let the children eat more, and his wife said: "Before this you helped the poor people. Now you are hungry, who will help you?" And Ying Fong said: "I see that my children are much smarter than common, and that makes me so happy that I forget my hunger; only it is hard for you to stand being hungry, and I am sorry for you." And his wife laughed and said: "I was only talking fun for you. You can be happy even in hard times. I am very glad that you can, and I am happy too."

While they were still speaking the sun shone, and Ying Fong went to the stony field to find some wild vegetables to eat, and he saw his stony ground full of lily bulbs. At that time he had never seen this kind of flower before, and did not know what kind it was. So he took plenty of the bulbs to carry home, and told his wife to try to cook them. But his wife said: "You do not understand what kind of nature there is to that. You keep that and see what grows from it. It is not good to eat." Ying Fong started to find some wild vegetables again, but his wife said: "You need not go any more, for while you were gone away two friends came, whom you helped once before when they were sick, and now they have heard from you and understand that you are sick, and one of them has left some money for you to buy plenty of food and meat," and the whole family was happy.

A month afterward the lilies were blooming and fragrant, and all the family was speaking of the very curious flower, and then a little six-year-old girl came running very early one day, and said: "That is a sacred flower, and the God is very glad for your good conduct, and has given this flower as a present for you, and it will make you very rich, and also you will have everlasting happiness by and by when you die." And while she was still speaking many other children came and said the same. It seems that an angel made them say so, and many people came from all the country round about and many of them bought that kind of flower to celebrate the Happy New Year. So, after several years, it went all through China, and Ying Fong became very rich.

Now Ying Fong's brother, Ti Fong, had been keeping a store and had lost all his money, so that he had to sell all of his property, and one day Mrs. Ti Fong sent for her husband and said: "Your brother, Ying Fong, is a man of good conduct and the God loves him. We are of such bad conduct that the God will punish us." And Ti Fong answered: "I fear so, but I will change my conduct to do good acts so that I can get away from the punishment." And his wife said: "That is what I thought," and that night they laid awake all night talking about changing their conduct and doing good, and early next morning they went to Ying Fong and embraced him and wept bitterly, and said: "You do everything that is good; you will receive everlasting happiness, but we are sinners and surely will be punished; now you must find some way to save us." Then Ying Fong answered: "The ordinary man when he commits some sin does not say sin. Now you say that you are sinners and you understand your sin. That is a good thing, a very good thing. I cannot find a better way to tell you that you are good already." And Ti Fong said: "No; you must find something to teach me." Then Ying Fong could not answer him, but Mrs. Ying Fong said: "Shall I try one way to teach them?" And Ti Fong said: "I shall be very glad if you will say something to me." Then Mrs. Ying Fong said: "Long ago there was a holy man who taught his students to make a book, with many different things in it with regard to conduct, and many different teachings as to good acts and many about bad acts. They were divided into small, medium and great things. The small things were represented by the numbers 1, 2, 3, 4, 5; medium by 10, 20, etc., and the great by 100 or 200. This book was a Book of Good

Doctrine, and was called Gon-go-gaw. It makes different lessons for different treatments. One was how to treat the mother and father; one how the Emperor should treat his people, and how the people should treat him; another how the husband should treat his wife, and the wife the husband; another how to treat the brother and the sister; another how to treat the friend, the merchant, the proprietor, the servant, etc. He told the students to follow that book, and every night before going to bed to take a book and write out how many good acts in that day and how many bad acts in that day, and then perform worship before the God before going to bed. And the first year the bad things came to more than the good things, and the second year the bad and the good were equal, and the third year the good acts were more than the bad acts, and the holy man said, 'When the good acts are more than the bad acts, that becomes merit, and then you will get everlasting happiness in this way.' Now the book is all through the country and everybody knows that you can try."

Then Mrs. Ti Fong said: "That is a very good way; that is a new life for me," and she would like to perform worship before the God right away, and would like to commence that day to begin to follow that book, but Ying Fong said: "Man's duty is to do all good. We cannot call a partial doing merit. The holy man knows that, but this way makes easy steps for the beginner, and after that Ti Fong's conduct became very good. When he was bad he had been more bad than common, but when he was good he was more good than common, because he had the more power in his nature, and all the surrounding country afterward became Christian and the jail was empty all the time.

And after that Ying Fong prospered and his children and his children's children, for he had more than a thousand descendants after him.

And from these came many high judges and wise men, more than in any other country, and every year they divided the flower money. There was not one poor man among them; all were rich. Thus the goodness of one man brought him and his descendants for so long a time such great happiness.

REMARKS ON THE FOREGOING BY DR. FOO.

Such is the story of the Sacred Lily of China, which teaches us many lessons. When Cum Ying Fong, a poor man, helped the people he was so poor that he could not do much. How is it that the good acts of one man made the whole family to become happy, so that now more than one thousand descendants altogether receive benefit, besides their everlasting happiness in heaven? I am just talking of what people can see. It seems strange that the good acts of one man for a short time should bring so much benefit for a long time. But I think that the seed of happiness is like the seed of a fruit—like the apple, for instance. An apple seed is a very light thing, but in a single seed I can see many branches, many leaves, many flowers and much fruit. But if I talk of all these things in the seed everybody will laugh and say: "That man talks too big for that little seed; that man is crazy." But when I put that seed into the good ground I need not wait so long as ten years, when there is a fine young tree, and soon after there are many branches and many leaves, and nice fruit hangs upon the branches. Then, in a few years more, the branches and leaves are more plentiful, and there is more fruit, and the people who pass by that tree say: "That's a good apple;" the children love that tree, and say, "Good apples," and present those apples to their friends; their good friends say: "Oh, that's a good apple," and it is sold in the store, and the customers say, "Good apples." The tree not only furnishes fruit for me, but all the family is furnished, not only for a short time, but for many years, and they all remember when the seed was very small and not put into the ground. But afterward it produced so much fruit and was of much benefit. And I think that the seed of happiness is just the same, and I am willing that the educated man, who knows the way to happiness, should teach me and many different teachings as to good acts and many about bad acts.

INDEX.

A.

Abscesses, cancers, etc., cures	208
Abscesses, womb, bowels, cured	158
Advantages of Oriental medicine	106
Air in sleeping room	79
Anatomy, Chinese system of	121
Appendicitis, first principles of cure	283
Appendicitis, seed lodging theory	282
Appendicitis, suggestions for those fearing	278
Appendicitis, three forms	280
Appendicitis, testimonials of cures	283
Arrowroot	50
Arrowroot blanc mange	49
Asthma and bronchitis cured	196
Asthma, cause and cure	190
Asthma, testimonials of cures	193-197

B.

Back and chest exercise	83-85
Baffled the best doctors	262
Barley water	46
Bathing and rubbing	77
Beef juice, essence	47
Beef tea—with oatmeal	48
Biliousness and headache cured	157
Bills of fare, Nos. 1, 2 and 3	20-23

Body, composition of	58-63
Body, analogous to engine	62
Brain exercise	84
Brain fever and other ailments cured	245
Breathing exercise	78
Bright's disease, diet	37
Bronchitis and indigestion cured	231
Broth, chicken, mutton, veal	48
Broth, Scotch, beef	50
Burns and scalds, treatment	82

C.

Cancers, abscesses and similar diseases	208
Cancer of bowels cured	212
Cancer of breast cured	214
Catarrh cured	220, 288
Catarrh and lung trouble cured	222
Catarrh, piles, sore eyes, cured	249
Catarrhal deafness cured	222
Caution to patients	74
Chart of the twelve pulse	147
Chest exercise	83
Chills and fever	182
Chinese medical book, fac simile of page	142
Chronic sufferers, benefit	72
Cold and cough of two years, cured	175
Cold, difficulty of a cure of a	169
Cold, how to cure a	168
Colds, atmospheric influences	170
Colds, guard against	79
Colds, improper treatment aggravates	170
Colds, predisposition	169
Colds, try a rational remedy	171
College of Oriental Medicine	101-104
Cooking, some points on	51
Complication of disorders cured	250
Constipation, chronic, diet in	39
Constipation, remedy for	81
Consumption averted	206
Consumption and hemorrhages, twelve causes of	198

Consumptive cough cured 162
Cure of a famous artist 230

D.

Diseases, cause and origin of................................ 126
Diet in anaemia and chlorosis 36
Diet in acute rheumatism 40
Diet in Bright's disease...................................... 37
Diet in bronchitis and asthma................................. 36
Diet in certain diseases 29
Diet in chronic rheumatism.................................... 41
Diet in constipation 39
Diet in diabetes mellitus 41
Diet in diarrhoea 38
Diet in diphtheria 34
Diet in dyspepsia 38
Diet in eczema 39
Diet in fever cases 31
Diet in general suggestions 23
Diet in gonorrhea 37
Diet in health 56
Diet in hemorrhoids 39
Diet in influenza and la grippe............................... 34
Diet for leaness 40
Diet in malarial fevers 34
Diet in measles 34
Diet in obesity 40
Diet in pneumonia 36
Diet in quinsy 37
Diet in scarlet fever... 34
Diet in tonsilitis 37
Diet in tuberculosis 35
Diet in typhoid fever... 33
Difference between this system and others.................... 72
Digestion and nutrition 124
Diploma, Tom Foo Yuen's 88
Diphtheria attack avoided 252
Dishes for invalids 41
Drink, evils of... 269
Drink habit, diagnosis of..................................... 272
Drink habit, T. Foo Yuen's analysis of........................ 270

Drink, milk and cinnamon 48
Drink, as to things to.. 24
Drinks 22

E.

Eczema, discussion of.. 216
Eczema cured 219
Eggnog 49
Egg timbales 45
Eggs, to cook.. 45
Emotions, effects of the... 127
Exercises, easy, but useful.. 83
Exercise for the back 85
Exercise for the brain... 84
Exercise for the chest 83
Exercise for the eyes.. 83
Exercise for the heart 83
Exercise for the lungs... 84
Exercise for the nerves 84
Exercise for the nerves and pulse 83
Exercise for the stomach and assist digestion........................ 83
Exercise the stomach and lower extremities.......................... 84
Eye, cataract cured.. 268
Eye, diseases of the... 263
Eye, sight saved 266
Eye, speedy cure of.. 265
Eyes, sore, cured.. 249
Eye wash 82

F.

Fish, proper way to cook 56
Food, amount required by man 65
Food, best to use.. 67
Foods from China... 70
Foods of the future.. 69
Food, substances that can be used as................................. 64
Food, uses in human body... 56
Food values compared 68
Food value of tea.. 27
Fresh air in sleeping rooms.. 79
Functions of the five vital organs................................... 122

G.

Great benefits to Americans	105
Growing old early	183
Guard against colds	79

H.

Habit, the curse of	269
Hallowell, W. A., Jr., testimonial	229
Herbal remedies	135
Herbal remedies, action of	138
Herbal remedies for women	150
Herbal remedies prepared	137
Healing, four methods of	128
Heart	123
Heart and stomach trouble cured	233
Hemorrhages, notable cure of	202
Hendren, Mrs., testimonial of	251
Home, first in Los Angeles	113
Home, second in Los Angeles	114
How to keep well	237
Humphrey, Clara, story of	208

I.

Imperial Medical College	131
Information for patrons and inquirers	72
Injuries to bone cured	261
Inflammatory rheumatism cured	239-241
Introduction	5

K.

Kidneys	124
Kidney and bladder troubles cured	228
Kidney, liver and lung trouble relieved	203
Klondike, a voice from the	165

L.

La Grippe cures	174-175
Laws regulating the profession	132
Lemonade	47
Letter of a well-known business man	228
Lily of China, legend of the sacred	290

Lime water 49
Liquor habit considered 269
Liquor habit, no cases too severe......................... 274
Liquor habit, testimonial 273
Los Angeles, from a prominent citizen of................. 225
Loss of leg threatened, but cured......................... 261
Lung trouble cured 201

M.

Malaria and climate 183
Malaria, complications from 186
Malaria, typical cases 184
Malarial poisoning 180
Malarial poisoning, three forms of........................ 181
Meat, extracts 54
Medicine versus surgery 254
Medical history in China 129
Milk punch 49
Mitral stenosis relieved 235
Moody, G. W., testimonial 109
Morphine habit cured 224
Mulled wine 47
Mushes, nutritious way to prepare......................... 46

N.

Nervous prostration cured 163
Neuralgia cured 105, 244
Nutrition and digestion 124

O.

Oatmeal gruel 50
Operation spared in bone cancer........................... 267
Oriental Medical College................................... 104
Oriental medicine's advantages 106
Oriental medicine, concise discussion of.................. 236
Oriental medicine, some topics from 121
Oriental system, compared with others..................... 217
Otis, Mrs. Eliza A., testimonial 162

P.

Patients, caution to 74

Patient, from a distance 223
Paralysis cured 185, 188, 227
Patrons' general letter of confidence........................... 110
Physicians, lack of good ones in China........................ 133
Physician's experience 226
Piles, cause and cure 246
Piles and other troubles cured 249
Pimples removed 163
Pneumonia cured 176
Points to be observed 76
Protein defined 65
Pulse chart 147
Punch, milk 49

R.

Relief of a difficult case 242
Relieved by this system 232
Remarkable cure of spine 259
Remedies, some handy... 80
Remedies, herbal, how to secure 275
Rheumatic pain remedy 81
Rice and apple 43
Rice cream 43
Rice, directions for cooking 43
Rice gruel 42
Rice water 42
Rubbing and bathing 77
Rupture and other troubles cured 223

S.

Scalds and burns, treatment 82
Scrofula cured 227
Sciatica cured 241
Serious case made well 234
Shoulder dislocated relieved 260
Skin diseases, remedy for 81
Sleep, the question of 125
Sleeping room, fresh air in... 79
Spleen 123
Statement of a remarkable case 173

Steaming, the best way to cook meats.................................. 54
Stewing, some points on 53
Stomach ache cure 82
Stomach trouble cured 159, 179
Stricture relieved 215
Soups 54
System, convinced of the merits of the............................. 177

T.

Thirst to quench 81
Throat, cure of chronic sore 177
Throat troubles cured 253
Tom Foo Yuen's biography 92
Tom Foo Yuen, certificates......................................86-91
Tom Foo Yuen's diploma 88
Tom Foo Yuen, esteem for 187
Tom Foo Yuen, gifts to 275
Tom Foo Yuen, portrait of 92
Tom Foo Yuen, sketch of 87
Tom Leong certificates 119, 120
Tom Leong, portrait of 116
Tom Leong, sketch of 115
Treatment found beneficial 178
Typhoid fever testimonial 172

V.

Vermiform appendix, function of 279
Vivisection among the Chinese 139

W.

Wash for the eye 82
Werth, Mrs. M. D., testimonial 243
Whiskey hurts blood and brain 271
Wine, mulled 47
Womb trouble cured 158, 164
Women, diseases 150
Women, for the special benefit of................................. 167

www.ingramcontent.com/pod-product-compliance
Lightning Source LLC
Chambersburg PA
CBHW060210040326
40610CB00008B/818